MERCURY FREE

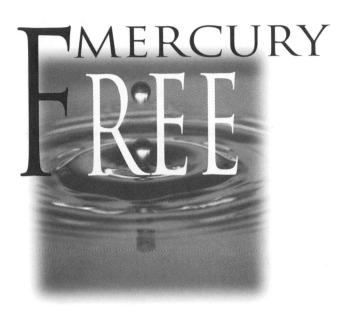

DR. JAMES E. HARDY

Dear Helyn ~

May you have great,
Success at all you do!

James Hardy

9·18·97 M

Title: Mercury-Free
Sub-Title: The wisdom behind the global consumer movement to ban "silver" dental fillings

Author: Dr. James E. Hardy

Copyright © 1996 by Dr. James E. Hardy

Publication Date: Autumn 1996
Hardcover Price $24.95 plus $3.95 shipping and handling ISBN: 0-9649301-1-0
Paperback edition Price $16.95 plus $3.95 shipping and handling ISBN: 0-9649301-0-2
Paperback Canada: Price $18.95 plus $4.95 shipping and handling
Finished size: 5-1/2" x 8-1/2"
Number of pages: 270
Publisher: Gabriel Rose Press, Inc.
Back matter: Index, bibliography
Address for Individual Orders: STCS Distributors • Box 246 • Dept. BK
                     Glassboro, NJ 08028-0246 • 1/800-266-5564 or FAX order
                     to (609) 881-8042
Publisher's Cataloging in Publication
(Prepared by Quality Books, Inc.)

Hardy, James E., 1952-
    Mercury-free: the wisdom behind the global consumer movement to ban "silver" dental
fillings / James E. Hardy.
    p. cm.
    Includes bibliographical references and index.
    ISBN 0-9649801-0-2

1. Mercury – Toxicology. 2. Dental amalgams – Toxicology. 3. Fillings (Dentistry) – Health
aspects. I. Title.

RA1231.M5H37 1996   615.9'25663
                         QBI96-40036

Acknowledgements

The whole idea behind healthcare is to seek the best possible method of treatment at all times. Change is natural and necessary. What has been done in the past is not always the best for the future. And hanging on to old ideas simply because of their age is unwise and unnatural. Truth seeks new understanding. As we progress through life it is up to each one of us to seek our own understanding of truth. The truth itself does not change, but our understanding of truth does.

May truth guide us in all we do. May this book contribute to your understanding of what is true. Since 1978, this book has grown from a seed planted in the garden of my mind to what you hold in your hand today. Lots of love and teamwork has allowed it to mature to its final form. Many talented and caring people have been responsible. First and foremost has been my friend, Mary. With her guidance, support and loving suggestions the book took shape. I am indeed fortunate to have such a partner.

I thank my brother Andrew for encouraging me to pursue this writing. He is loving, kind and gifted.

I respect and admire my friend Beth Hollenbeck. Her knowledge and dedication to environmental health is world-class. Thank you Beth for making this a better book through your suggestions.

Many other people have assisted in refining the text, making it more readable and understandable. My friends Gabriel Sheets, Suzan Goldin, Dana Wright, JoAnn Montilla all spent hours making excellent recommendations for clarity. Professional editing was provided by my respected friends, Lewis Rothlein and Beverly Dutton. Artistic genius was added to the cover and text design by Mickey Gill. Patricia Denninger's friendship, hard work and belief in me has also played an important role.

A special thank you goes to Bill Gurvitch. He is one of those rare individuals who is willing to share his expertise just because he believes in the future of mankind. He truly wants others to succeed in making this a better world.

To all those who made this book possible, I thank you with all my being.

Author's note

Mercury-Free is intended to provide you with information you can use to supplement, not replace conventional medical care. If you have health challenges, consult with your physician before making any changes suggested by this book.

Everyone is unique in how they are able to tolerate exposure to different metals and chemicals. Not everyone will respond the same way to mercury amalgam removal. Some may benefit greatly, some may not. It depends on many factors. It is therefore advisable to consult with your physician on these matters prior to beginning any amalgam removal or mercury detoxification program.

The latest medical research has provided the basis of the information in this book. But science is always moving forward and new developments occur over time. Future research findings may alter the recommendations contained within this book.

I intend this book to be a reference to those who want to be educated dental consumers. It is my hope that it will strengthen dentist-patient and physician-patient relationships by creating meaningful dialog. Share the information with your dentist and physician so that you can all work together as a team in more abundant health and happiness.

I owe a debt of gratitude to many people during the birth process

Dedication

of <u>Mercury-Free.</u> However, the reason I wrote this book is to make our planet a better place for us and our children. Our sons and daughters are the caretakers of tomorrow. We owe them our best. So, it is with great love and joy I dedicate this book to my children, Forrest Gabriel and Summers Rose.

INTRODUCTION

While mercury has been used in dental "silver" fillings for over 160 years, its use has always been filled with controversy. There has never been a dental filling material so long used and so long opposed. Even when it was introduced to the United States in 1834, physicians called its use in fillings malpractice. This obsolete, unhealthy, inferior and ugly filling, the mercury amalgam, is still with us. However, its retirement is drawing near.

Mercury is dangerous, more poisonous than lead or arsenic. Everyone's dental "silver" amalgams are composed of mostly mercury. They release mercury vapor into the body 24 hours a day. And, although more than a dozen new filling materials have been shown to be superior to silver-mercury amalgam, it is still the most often used material in dentistry. Today, there is overwhelming evidence that using mercury fillings in dentistry is second-rate at best, extremely toxic at worst. Because of the threat mercury poses to our health and the health of our planet, it clearly has no place in the future of dentistry.

In August 1981 I spent some time in the Arizona Hopi and Navajo reservations. One crisp, cloudless, moonless night in the desert, I lay down among the cacti, looked up and saw something new. There were many more planets and stars filling the heavens than I had ever seen. Each had a different size and brightness. In truth, the sky was the clearest and the night the darkest I had ever experienced, so I was able to see more of what was always there. I lay there for a long time, awed by the newness of this night sky. Now I look up at night and remember all that I saw. Even when the stars and planets are not all visible to me, I know they are there.

The intent of <u>Mercury-Free</u> is to clear the air for you, so that you will know how much information has always been out there against the continued use of mercury in dentistry. I want this book to remove the haze, the smog, the clouds and the man-made lights, so you can see a clear picture of what is true, as clear as the sky I saw that night in the desert. My hope is that once you've read this book, you will never feel the same about "silver" fillings.

The title has dual meaning. Mercury, in Roman mythology, is a messenger or guide. <u>Mercury-Free</u> is intended to be a guide to help you make informed, intelligent and appropriate choices about dentistry. And it will reveal many messages on the nature of mercury and how it adversely affects us and our planet.

Mercury as a planet is the hottest in our solar system. Mercury as an issue has been the hottest one ever in dentistry. <u>Mercury-Free</u> intends to turn up the heat so that dentistry rids itself of mercury amalgam, the nineteenth century blunder.

If we respect and love ourselves and our environment, we will not allow the continued use of mercury in our teeth. Beauty certainly dictates that fillings be the same natural color as our teeth; the strong, relatively new composite resin fillings match natural colors. On the other hand, mercury amalgams are at first a harsh metallic-silver color and later turn a crusty black. In addition to amalgam's ugliness in appearance, it is also ugly to your well-being. Mercury amalgam is dangerous because it releases toxic mercury into the body. Mercury may cause chronic fatigue, migraine headaches, MS-like symptoms, arthritis-like joint pain, personality and behavioral disorders, kidney failure, brain damage and birth defects. There are as many as 200 symptoms listed in the medical literature for mercury poisoning. Mercury poisoning can happen with one large dose of mercury or constant small doses, as in the case of dental amalgams.

I love being a dentist. I enjoy my profession even more now

than when I started. The reason is that I know I'm having a positive impact on people's lives. It seems as though every day I'm getting wonderful feedback from my patients. They have less arthritic pain, more stamina, and they feel happier and think more clearly. In short, their quality of life is better because they have chosen to be mercury-free. This encourages me to stand up for what I believe to be true: dental mercury amalgams are making people sick. That is why I wrote this book.

We the consumers would be wise if we refused mercury. Greed, false pride and ignorance on the part of the powerful dental interests foster an unwillingness to forgo the use of mercury amalgam. But, if we don't buy mercury, it won't be sold. Our personal and environmental health and safety must come first.

Earth is our home. It represents our larger body. What we do to the Earth will always come back to us. So many people are understanding this basic truth today that there is an explosion of interest and knowledge about our environment. In this book, I explore the environmental consequences of using mercury in dentistry and other industries. I urge you to read my book, tell others what you've read and take action. Take action not only for yourself, but also for the world our children will inherit. You and I are the caretakers of tomorrow.

This book, then, is about the long and controversial use of mercury in dentistry. It is about loving ourselves and loving our planet. This book is about being

Mercury-Free.

TABLE OF CONTENTS

Symptoms of Mercury Poisoning include:

- Arthritis-like joint pain
- Asthma
- Amyotrophic Lateral Sclerosis
- Antibiotic Resistance
- Abnormal Hunger
- Anorexia Nervosa
- Birth Defects
- Candidiasis (yeast infection)
- Cerebral Palsy
- Chronic Fatigue
- Diabetes Insipidus-like symptoms
- Epstein-Barr infection
- Food Hypersensitivities
- Graves Disease-like symptoms
- Hearing disturbances
- Heart Attacks
- Hyperglycemia
- Immune system imbalances
- Menstrual Disturbances
- Migraine Headaches
- MS-like symptoms
- Oral Diseases
- Parkinson's Disease-like symptoms
- Tremors
- Vision Disturbances

Chapter 5

- Experts agree that mercury fillings are the largest source of environmental mercury exposure in humans.
- How amalgam killed four in Michigan.
- Kids' toys and shoes may contain mercury.
- Why your dentist's office may not be safe.
- How mercury from amalgam pollutes our water, air and soil.
- How dental mercury use contributes to global atmospheric pollution.
- Why the world's largest case of environmental mercury pollution comes from dental mercury.
- Previous disasters from mercury pollution that forewarn us.
- How the U.S. bans mercury in paint and pesticides, but not in fillings or vaccines.
- Burning issues: pollution from the living.
- Burning issues: pollution from the dead.
- The politics of amalgam.
- Good news: amalgam banned in other countries and water is being cleaned up.

Chapter 6

- A brief review of the book.
- Practical advice on what you can do about mercury use in your dentist's office and your body.
- An important choice: How you can become mercury-free.

1

Chapter 1: "I Wanted To Graduate"

becoming

aware

I Wanted
to Graduate

Grandma's tea set and the Lone Ranger

When I was ten, I went to the dentist for a filling. I remember sitting in a pale green, vinyl dental chair. The silver-haired doctor in his white coat told me that he would fix my cavity with a nice "silver" filling. That sounded good. Images of grandma's tea set and shiny silverware on her mahogany dining table drifted through my mind.

Oddly enough, I found myself thinking of my favorite TV show, "The Lone Ranger." His white horse was named Silver. The phrase I remember him best for was, "Hi-Oh Silver, away!" Whenever I hear the William Tell overture, I can still see Silver raising up on his back legs, with the Lone Ranger waving, his hat in his hand.

All these images were comforting to me and I believed my dentist would give me a silver filling as pure as my grandmother's tea set. I trusted my dentist like I trusted the Lone Ranger.

The truth about "silver" fillings

I didn't find out what was really in my silver fillings until I was a 26-year-old freshman dental student at Washington University in St. Louis. Silver fillings are not really silver fillings at all. They are composed mostly of mercury. "Silver" fillings contain up to 70% mercury and as little as 20% silver.

Other metals commonly used in fillings are tin, copper and zinc. Silver-mercury fillings are called amalgams by the dental profession, because they are an amalgam, or mixture, of mercury and other metals.[1] Webster's unabridged dictionary defines "amalgam" as any metallic alloy of which mercury is an essential part. Given the enormous quantity of mercury, silver fillings could well be called mercury fillings.

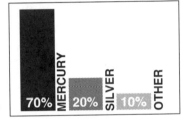

I was curious, but I wanted to graduate

It was in a dental materials class that I learned amalgam fillings have up to 700,000 parts per million mercury. I was stunned. I knew at the time that the FDA took tuna fish off our grocery shelves when it had only 1 part per million mercury. So, raising my hand, I asked the professor, "Given the fact that our government removes tuna fish from stores with only 1 part per million mercury, how is it remotely safe to put 700,000 times this concentration in our patients' teeth and allow them to chew on it for years?" (I recalled reading about the Minamata Bay disaster in Japan. The people there ate fish containing mercury and there were an unusually high number of birth defects, mental retardations, cerebral palsies and premature deaths.)

Chapter 1

It was not a popular question with my teacher. He answered me defensively:

"The mercury is all locked up in the filling and does not escape." I then asked, "If the mercury is all locked up, why do amalgams crack, break and completely wear out, needing replacement?" By the look on his face, this question was even less well received. He said, "Since the mouth is the harshest environment for any material, no material is considered permanent." He spoke of temperature extremes in the mouth, changing salt concentrations, tremendous compressive and grinding pressures exerted thousands of times per day during meals or any time the mouth was used.

He never gave me a straight answer about why he believed mercury was safe. And I felt the irritation in his voice growing. If anything, he made me even more curious as to why dentists would want to use mercury alloy in such harsh circumstances. I was even pulled aside after class by some of my classmates and told that I was a good student but "don't blow it by asking so many questions about mercury." I was curious but wanted to graduate. I knew I could rock the boat only so far, as I was in it, so I decided two things:

1. Not to ask any more pointed questions regarding mercury.
2. To do my own research and find out my own answers.

Questioning the status quo and voicing dissent in the dental profession can be met with intimidation, harassment and character assassination. To date, there have been at least four dentists in the U.S. forced to close their practices because of their positions on the use of mercury amalgam.[2]

The claim by the ADA that mercury amalgam is safe is, in my opinion and that of countless others, untrue. However, the large majority of dentists and dental politicos seem to be content to nod in unison with this position.

Freshman versus the establishment

Here I was, questioning amalgam, the very material for which the "Grand Old Man of Dentistry," G.V. Black, was best known. In 1978 I was just a freshman student in the same school that had G. V. Black as a lecturer in 1870. Next to Pierre Fauchard, called the "Father of Dentistry," G. V. Black is the most highly respected dentist in all of history. Black was born on August 3, 1836, a full 25 years before the American Civil War. Much of his extensive work on amalgam, written over 100 years ago, is still taught to dental students throughout the world today. Spending his later years in Chicago, Black died in 1915 and a monument was even erected for him in one of the windy city's parks.[3] Given all the advancements during the last 100 years in the related fields of science and medicine, is dentistry keeping current by using such old techniques and technology as amalgam?

Worldwide search

I decided to take my questions about mercury to the library. So, after class, I requested a Medline computer search to find all the research containing the word "mercury" from the turn of the century up till that day, in all available languages. A Medline search looks through all medical literature printed and referenced by the Library of Congress. Hundreds of abstracts were found, and I read through them all. Some articles were in Russian, German, French and other foreign languages.

Fortunately for me, many patients that came to the dental school were immigrants who lived in ethnic neighborhoods. They spoke many different languages. I was able to have every single article translated into English through my patients' kindness and generosity.

In all those documents, there was virtually no positive news about mercury. Nearly all the books and articles painted a grim picture of mercury's negative impact on human health and our environment. Hundreds of articles said the same thing: mercury, even in tiny amounts, was poisonous. It was confirmed and reconfirmed to be harmful to almost every system in the human body as well as our larger body, the environment.

To make things worse, symptoms of mercury poisoning are very often misdiagnosed for months or even, tragically, for years.[4] The main reasons for the misdiagnoses are: one, the medical profession's unfamiliarity with the disease, and two, the unique way symptoms are expressed from person to person.

Vague symptoms

In cases of long-term low-level mercury poisoning, the onset of symptoms may be delayed for years. This is the type of mercury exposure one receives from amalgams.

Initial mercury poisoning symptoms may include vague psychological and behavioral disturbances such as short term memory loss, mood swings, anxiety, depression, fits of anger, irritability, indecision, excitability, shyness, fatigue, headaches, nightmares or more severe personality disorders. Long-term, low-level exposure to mercury can slow reaction times and decrease ability to perform delicate tasks.[5,6,7,8,9,10]

These are problems I certainly do not want in my body or in my dentist's body. Because these signs of poisoning can happen slowly, over such a long time, very few people would suspect their nice "silver" fillings, put in 20 years prior. How could they be the source of such symptoms? At first glance, it may seem far-fetched. But when one gives dental mercury a closer look, it makes sense.

It is not unusual for people to have their first mercury amalgam filling at around nine years of age. The first amalgam begins their life-long exposure to mercury vapor. Mercury is released from the surface of amalgams in the form of vapor. As people age, the chance of receiving more amalgams increases. The more amalgams one has, the more the exposure to mercury vapor. Many people with amalgam fillings have had them most of their lives, so they are receiving what is called long-term, or chronic exposure to mercury from their fillings.

Chronic mercury exposure is cumulative. It builds up in the brain, kidneys and other vital tissues. This kind of mercury exposure is more insidious and difficult to trace than one large dose called acute mercury exposure. As a result, chronic mercury vapor exposure can be even more dangerous than a walloping one-dose exposure.

I've often heard people say, "I've had amalgams for 25 years, and I don't feel anything." Well, it is nearly impossible to determine how one might feel without a toxin if it has been part of one's life for so long.

Many of my patients have requested amalgam removal for cosmetic reasons or as a hedge against future mercury-related problems. They did not sense any ill effects from having amalgams for 25 years. But, when the amalgams were replaced, a large percentage of these same people noticed unexpected health improvements. For example, they said their memory improved or their thinking felt clearer, more precise. And some noticed having more energy and stamina, or experiencing more calmness and a greater sense of well-being.

I wanted to graduate, so I did my own research and made up my own mind not to use mercury when I became a licensed dentist. Today, my wish is for the entire dental profession to finally graduate from the use of mercury to the stronger, safer, healthier, alternative fillings, composite resins.

The following chapter deals with real people's stories who, after becoming mercury-free, went from sickness to health.

2

Chapter 2: From Sickness to Health

filled with

hope

From Sickness to Health

Dr. Hardy's health-centered dentistry

My practice has evolved from just mercury-free dentistry to health-centered dentistry. Let me explain. When I began dental practice, I was committed to being mercury-free. Over the years of interacting with my knowledgeable and wonderful patients, I have learned that being mercury-free is only a part of what I envision as whole-person or health-centered dentistry. My patients have taught me that the bigger picture matters in order to deliver the best possible dentistry. The bigger picture involves knowing about patients' eating and living habits. It involves knowing about the balance of stress and fun in their lives. It also involves a general picture of the emotions each patient brings into my office.

I have never seen a set of teeth walk into my office without a body attached. I've never seen someone walk into my office without emotional attachments. And I've never seen someone with poor eating habits and a stressful lifestyle who didn't eventually manifest physical consequences.

So in my practice of health-centered dentistry, I learn as much as I can about the patients, then share what I know about the interrelationships of physical, emotional and dental health. This information allows me to be a better dentist.

For example sugar or corn syrup in soft drinks or other food and nicotine and caffeine, tend to promote gum disease or decay. High stress, anxiety or depression can promote gum disease, canker sores, and decay by lessening a person's willingness to take proper care of his or her mouth. A poor diet can create stress as easily as a high pressure job.

We have different paths in life that create different tastes. That's why they make more flavors than chocolate and vanilla. So, I believe each patient is an individual with individual needs. How I treat patients depends on the bigger picture of who they are, not just what their teeth look like.

At my office, I see my patients as whole persons, complex and original. In the heart of my office philosophy rests their good health.

A Package Deal

Good health is a package deal. Emotions are connected to the body. The thigh bone is connected to the knee bone. And "all them bones" carry a person around who has feelings, emotions and desires. Humans are package deals.

I called one of my patient's physicians recently to ask whether she had any heart murmur. The nurse on the phone said, "Oh, we don't have anything to do with her heart, we only treat the ulcers on her legs." I asked if there was any medical history on the patient. She proudly said, "Yes, we have 20 years' worth." I asked if there was any

11

indication in that 20-year history of any heart murmur, she said "No, but we have nothing to do with her heart." Well, I beg to differ.

Her heart has been with her on every office visit, and I dare say will continue to come in every time her legs visit. You see, too often this is the prevailing medical attitude: "It's not my specialty, so I don't deal with it." Wrong! If anyone deals with anyone, they deal with the whole package, not a collection of parts or specialties. As a dentist, I don't just look at my patient's teeth and gums. Good dental health is also a package deal. There are many good ways of knowing the whole patient.

In my practice, I approach each patient from a perspective of balance. When a new patient comes in for an examination, I ask questions designed to give me a picture of not just their dental health, but their overall health. I listen for how they reply as well as what they say. This way I get a picture of where the balance is in their lives. I ask questions such as:

How would you rate your refined sugar intake? From what sources do you get the sugar?

What is your caffeine intake? From what sources?

Do you eat many vegetables?

Do you eat many green salads?

Do you eat much fruit?

Do you eat much protein? From what sources?

Do you eat many complex carbohydrates?

Do you eat much fat? From what sources?

Do you chew gum? How much?

Do you chew ice?

Do you exercise? What kind? How often?

Do you drink alcohol? How much?

Do you have much stress? From what sources?

Do you have much fun?

Patients almost always say, "FUN?" Yes, fun is whatever puts happiness in our lives, so this is one of the most important questions. If

fun does not balance at least equally with stress, there is a problem.
**Do you smoke? How much? How long? Do you plan to quit?
Do you find time for yourself? If not, why?
Do you sleep well? If not, why?
Do you have any eating disorders of which you are aware?
If so, how long? Are you seeking help?**

Sick teeth

I have had the pleasure of talking about dental amalgam to a variety of groups -- parents, spouses, businesspersons, social workers, physicians, dentists, psychologists, engineers, toxicologists, university students and retirees. Most have responded with interest because nearly everyone has some teeth which are filled with mercury amalgam.

After one talk to a group of retirees, an 80-year-old woman came up to me and relayed the following story. Her grandfather had been a dentist in the hills of western North Carolina. He told her it was common in the late 1800s for the physicians of very sick patients who didn't respond to any other treatment to have all the patient's teeth extracted. Some patients would get better after their teeth were gone. No one knew why, but it helped.

She said, "I'll bet taking out the mercury with the extracted teeth was the reason they got better." She wished her grandfather was still alive today so he could hear this.

Thousands of people across the world have had their mercury fillings removed and replaced with composites and have seen their sicknesses dramatically improve or even disappear -- people with symptoms of multiple sclerosis, arthritis, lupus, candida (yeast), chronic fatigue, depression, anxiety, memory loss, headaches, colitis and Alzheimer's.

You are about to read the stories of people with various illnesses, often misdiagnosed or tossed off as neuroses, that just happened to

13

get better, by replacing their amalgam fillings with composite resins. I believe that getting better from an illness usually involves more than one change. Sometimes, however, making just one change turns the tide from sickness to health.

Letters from patients

Dear Dr. Hardy, and all who are concerned,

I wish to share with you the changes within me, physically, as well as psychologically, since you removed all my old mercury fillings. I was plagued with headaches all my life, for as long as I can remember. I had no resistance to infection. I had earaches. My body failed to respond to diets . . . I spent years studying nutrition and diet . . . All these self treatments would bring just limited results. I just never felt very well . . .

I had all my fillings replaced . . . After five years of no mercury poisoning . . . The headaches are nearly gone . . . After Dr. Hardy [removed the mercury], my body began to respond to diets, to metabolize and to heal itself. My eyesight even improved. My skin became more radiant . . . I do not contract colds or flu like I used to. When I do, I heal much faster. My self-image has greatly improved. I feel younger and I have much more ambition . . .

I definitely attribute all these positive changes to the removal of mercury, and a continued mercury-free oral care and maintenance program . . .

Dr. Hardy, thank you for giving me back my health and my life.

Rev. Carol Jo Garfinkel
Florida

Dear Dr. Hardy,

I have, or should I say, am being released from spasmatic muscular MS (Multiple Sclerosis). After six years of conventional medical treatment, ACTH, pain killers, muscle relaxants, anti-clotting medications, etc. I had had it with drug therapy . . .

It took a month and a half to remove 13 fillings. I am astonished at the changes that took place even in the chair. The first reaction [was] for the kidneys to kick in making it necessary to make a trip down the hall. Another immediate difference was a clearing in my head. I no longer feel as if I am living in a fog. As each removal was done this improved tremendously. The ability to think and concentrate after years of "vagueness" was terrific! One real blessing is a feeling of being interested in life and in doing things again. My energy level is also way up. The physical improvements are noticeable but the changes in my mental and emotional states [have] been outstanding!

I have been on a nutritional program for seven months which has included a chiropractor, a dentist (which also involved a TMJ adjustment), and a cranial osteopath. I feel I am about 60-70% recovered from this painful disease.

It is truly a miracle that these answers to such suffering are available. I have to be honest and say that it takes total commitment and that the road has not been an easy one but, without exception, absolutely worth it.

I sent along a list of symptoms [that have improved]. Perhaps it will be a help to someone. Here are a few of my worst:

Headaches for years - especially upon arising every morning
Extreme fatigue
High pitch noises in the ears
Muscle spasms in the legs, back and throat - choking
Disinterest in life, a feeling of withdrawing from people

Insomnia
Tremors, "electricity" especially in heat
Speech difficulties
Vision problems, blurring, cloudy
Pain in the spinal cord, hot spots
Non-specific pain anywhere in the body

Patricia Patterson
Pennsylvania

Dear Doctor Hardy,

I was raised on a farm in eastern Colorado. My grandfather, father and uncle raised wheat, and kept dairy cattle. Most of the seed was coated with mercury [fungicide-pesticide].

When I was 4, I fell and cut my left knee. It was a deep cut, several inches long. My father literally poured mercurochrome on this wound; mercurochrome didn't "burn" so I didn't cry when my father poured the purple liquid all over my knee. (mercurochrome contains mercury) Later, when I was unable to walk and suffering from painful joints, mercury poisoning was not diagnosed.

I was admitted to Children's Hospital in Denver, Colorado, and a diagnosis was never reached other than a possible side effect of penicillin, or rheumatoid arthritis.

When I was 11 or 12, a small mercury (amalgam) filling was placed in a molar; I didn't have a cavity; it was a preventative measure. I don't recall being sick then, but throughout adolescence, I was extremely depressed, and I developed a terrible sense of balance.

When I was 17, I attended a training school to become a medical assistant. About halfway into this schooling, I became very fatigued, barely able to get out of bed. I also experienced numerous "aches and pains", including chest pains and difficulty breathing. The doctor . . . gave me vitamin C, intravenously, in his office. I was well within a week and continued school.

In December of 1973, my daughter Becky was born. I was 24. In the year following her birth, I was extremely fatigued and experienced numbness and tingling sensations. I 'diagnosed' myself, and told my husband I thought I had MS. Then I became pregnant with our son, Tom. I was sick the entire pregnancy; 4 months into the pregnancy I experienced visual disturbances. I was immediately diagnosed with toxemia, and spent the next four months in bed. I was hospitalized four times during this pregnancy; to my knowledge, the highest my blood pressure ever was was 140/90, and even though several 24 hour urine tests were done, toxemia could not be confirmed.

My third pregnancy was a repeat of the second, except I voluntarily went to bed. Following this pregnancy, I experienced hemorrhaging: I took birth control pills to try to control this and [had] several MS attacks, which were blamed on the birth control pills. In August of 1977, I had a hysterectomy, and I also had my first two cavities filled with mercury. I 're-diagnosed' myself as having MS several times in the following years, but it was not officially diagnosed by a doctor until 1981.

When I had my next cavity filled in 1985, I asked for a composite [a mercury-free resin filling]. I knew nothing of the mercury amalgam debate, it was just a casual choice. The dentist accused me of being 'vain,' and said I would have to make a new appointment. It took no less than three hours for him to place one composite filling. He also decided to cover over the small amalgam filling; he told me he had drilled it partially out and covered it over with composite as I was leaving. This man knew I had MS, and I believe he was being facetious; in retrospect I realize that his comments were made in light of his knowledge of the "amalgam war" that I knew nothing of.

17

That afternoon I experienced one of the worst MS attacks I ever had. My legs were weak and I walked only with help. I remembered that this was what it was like when I was four years old. Sensory feelings were so distorted that everything that touched me below my waist was excruciatingly painful. The doctor assumed I probably had a bladder infection (no culture was done) and put me on Bactrium. This induced an allergic reaction of giant uticaria [hives], on my already super-sensitive skin. (Since mercury is mined with sulfa, no one will convince me that my body wasn't reacting to sulfa and mercury in different ways). I partially recovered from this attack, but my health went downhill in the following years.

Then I read the October 15, 1990 issue of *Newsweek* about "Toxic Teeth." The next day my husband and I went to the library and researched mercury poisoning. We read several books, and with Dr. Joyal Taylor's book in hand, I went to our dentist and asked him to remove the mercury fillings following Dr. Taylor's suggestions. On November 7 and November 20, 1990, the fillings were removed. In spite of a rubber dam and breathing oxygen [safeguards against mercury exposure during amalgam removal], I experienced MS symptoms several hours after the first appointment. I think this was partially due to a loose fitting oxygen mask; since I could smell the rubber of the rubber dam, some mercury vapor could have gotten through. Following the second appointment, I took a 5 mg. tablet of Xanax and went to bed. Since even 2.5 mgs. of Xanax will "knock me out", I remember very little of that night. However, there were no symptoms the next day.

Three days after the fillings were removed, the fatigue I knew so well was nearly gone. Most of the sensory disturbances left from 1985 were gone within six months. I used to get painful 'electric shocks' down my legs; I felt like I was plugged into a wall socket. Now I only have a slight tingling when I am extremely tired or emotionally upset. Also, the blind spots in my vision were gone in six months. My balance was greatly improved within several weeks of amalgam removal; I could not walk more than ten feet without falling or losing my balance, now I walk around a college campus. And the list goes on, and on.

But, I'm not "home free," by any means. In December of 1992, I became totally blind in my right eye following exposure to mercury from paint, a flu shot and a tetanus shot. I have learned that I cannot be too cautious -- mercury could be in anything. MS is not an acronym that represents a disease, in my opinion, but stands for Mercury Sensitivity, or Mercury Syndrome. I believe that mercury poisoning is responsible for all of the sickness I have related to you. I have thought about writing a "new book" (I, of course, have not written one book) and titling it The REAL Quacks Belong To The Dental/Medical Association.

Everything I shared with you can be verified by medical/dental records.

Kathleen Harner
Florida

Let's look at some areas of concern brought forth by Kathleen's letter. First, placing a composite filling should only take a few minutes more than an amalgam. The three hours she endured having one composite put in was unbelievably slow dentistry.

Mercury compounds are used as fungicides and pesticides to treat seeds intended for planting. Handling these seeds and breathing the fungicides or pesticides can be dangerous. Merthiolate and Mercurochrome were mercury compounds used as topical antiseptics. The FDA concluded in 1982 that they were ineffective and unsafe.[11]

Mercury compounds are still used in many vaccines as preservatives. Each dose of DPT, for example, contains thimerosal, the chemical name for Merthiolate.[12,13]

There are reports in the scientific literature of humans exposed to

19

mercury vapor developing diffuse red and itchy skin rashes.[14,15] Inorganic mercury exposure in humans has been reported to cause itchy measles-like spots, fever, mouth inflammation and a red rash all over the face and body.[16] The next letter describes these very same symptoms in a 14-year-old boy.

Dear Sir,

Our 14 year-old son, Francis T. Kuehl, D.O.B: 12-20-71, we believe is . . . [sensitive] to mercury. For about three years, our son had severe skin rashes for no apparent reason. His lower legs and feet broke out in rashes and deep skin cracks. These cracks would be deep enough to bleed and would be from 1/2 to 3 inches long. He was just miserable. This went on for several years. His baby teeth were full of amalgam, including a crown over amalgam. We had numerous visits with doctors and skin specialists, but no one found any reason for the rashes. At times he was so sore it was hard to walk. When his last baby tooth fell out, this was the crown over amalgam, all of the problems he had cleared up. About six months later we learned there was mercury in amalgam fillings.

His skin rash returned only two times since. He has never had, nor will he ever have amalgam in his permanent teeth. His skin rash returned a day after eating fresh seafood from the Pacific Ocean. This lasted two weeks. He ate seafood (fresh salmon) a second time from the Pacific Ocean. The following day the rash returned and an allergist had to be consulted because the rash was so bad he couldn't get rid of it. I phoned the local Fish and Game biologist and was told the ocean fish in this area contain small amounts of mercury.

The allergist ran tests and our son showed no allergic reaction to any fish, including the one he ate. The only time he had the rashes was when he had amalgam in his mouth or came into contact with items or food known to contain mercury.

During the time his baby teeth had amalgams, he never got rid of the rash.

When we talked to the allergist about the rash on my son, it was as if he didn't believe us. He told us that mercury was very low on his list and did not want to run tests for that.

It irritates me to no end when you tell a doctor what you have observed and he, in so many words, tells you that you are a liar, especially when you know what your kids eat or come into contact with . . . You tell them just . . . to protect yourself to avoid medications with mercury-based preservatives. Some doctors look at you like you're nuts or say there is so little in this, it won't hurt you.

The only way we found we [were] able to avoid medications with mercury-based preservatives was to hand deliver a letter to hospitals and doctors about [his] reaction to mercury. This then woke them up like "here comes a lawsuit" if [they] use it.

Franklin V. Kuehl
California

Note: How unfortunate that this parent felt he had to nearly threaten a lawsuit to protect his son from further mercury poisoning. Mercury has been removed from interior latex paint, so parents can feel safe about the paint they put on the walls of the nursery. How wonderful it will be to know parents can feel safe about dental fillings again when the fillings they allow in their children's mouths don't contain mercury.

The next letter was written to a support group for people with Chronic Epstein-Barr Virus, also called Chronic Fatigue Syndrome (CFS). An article in The *Harvard Medical School Health Letter* of May 1985, points out that the Epstein-Barr virus (the virus that causes mononucleosis) has been found to be a factor in a few cases of CFS. The article describes CFS symptoms as slight to debilitating fatigue, headaches, aches in muscles and joints, sore throat, swollen lymph nodes, and low-grade fever. Periods of sickness may continue on and off for years. One lady, 48, had CFS symptoms for 17 years. The article noted that some CFS patients had no previous history of mononucleosis.

The *Harvard Medical School Health Letter* article ends by saying that even if one finds out through the proper blood test that he or she has a lingering infection from Epstein-Barr virus, an effective treatment is not available.[17]

CFS has also been said to be caused by the new rubella vaccine. This vaccine was introduced in 1979. CFS was first reported in the U.S. in 1982. Peripheral nerve pain, numbness, and paralysis, along with joint pain and arthritis are side effects caused by the vaccine.[18]

Routine examinations of undiagnosed patients are often inconclusive. When nothing can be found on standard tests, people with chronic fatigue are often thought to be neurotic.

The causes of CFS seem to be multifactorial. What is known is that people who have CFS should not be exposed to mercury. Mercury suppresses the human immune system. Is some CFS caused by exposure to mercury? How much do amalgams worsen CFS? I have seen several of my own patients with chronic fatigue find blessed relief after becoming mercury-free.

The following letter details the story of a young man who suffered from chronic fatigue.

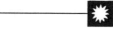

Dear Kris,

Thank you for sending me all the information re: CEBV support group. I am sending you a packet sent to me by Dr. James Hardy, one of the pioneering dentists in the field of mercury-free dentistry.

During the period from July 28, 1983 until September 1985, I experienced the most bizarre set of symptoms one could experience. After 12 trips to doctors, nutritionists and related health professionals, it was not until August 13, 1985, after having four amalgam mercury-silver fillings removed that I began to notice improvements. Gradually, the wide range of symptoms that I experienced began to disappear.

At the time, I had no idea that anyone else could possibly have a similar set of symptoms. But when a good friend in Los Angeles sent me the article about your research in the *Los Angeles Times,* a gut feeling told me to check into the possibility that I might have somehow contracted a virus unknown to the diagnostic tools available to the health professionals that I visited.

Now, after receiving your "Sign-symptom complex consistent with CEBV [Chronic Epstein-Barr Virus] syndrome" list, I am almost completely sure that I had a real illness, that it wasn't "just in your mind" as I'm sure many of your support people have been told.

I had the following set of symptoms which did not go away for two years!!

1. FATIGUE (Severe most of the time -- as if I had mild mononucleosis for two years straight.) (I had been a competitive athlete previously!)

2. FREQUENT SORE THROATS & COLDS Despite a healthy diet, no smoking, no sugar, no alcohol.

3. COGNITIVE FUNCTION PROBLEMS These were the most noticeable and the most frightening to me. I had just completed a rigorous master's degree program at USC and never had any lapses in thought. All of a sudden, I would forget large blocks of short term memory . . . I would put something down, look away, and then actually forget where it was! ! ! I couldn't concentrate. I would find myself having trouble with depth perception which affected my vision. And most frightening of all, I found myself unable to say what I wanted to in an articulate manner. I would think, "Hello how are you?" and I would end up saying, "Hello, how . . ." and the words wouldn't come

out or they would come out backwards or in nonsensical sounds. I thought I had some sort of neurological damage.

4. PSYCHOLOGICAL PROBLEMS (1983-1984) I experienced, for the first time in my life, terrible panic attacks (a low blood sugar diet drastically reduced them throughout 1984 & 1985!) which lasted 15 to 30 seconds, five to eight times a day. I really thought I was going crazy. I had always been a very strong person emotionally, and was never the type of person to break down and cry. I experienced low-grade anxiety for nearly a full year after I first experienced the symptoms.

5. CNS [CENTRAL NERVOUS SYSTEM] EFFECTS Cluster headaches -- left side of head and eye-Visual disturbances -- July 1985, I lost all vision in left eye for 30 minutes -- eye doctor found nothing wrong. -Extreme sensitivity to bright light. This didn't go away until 30 days after my mercury fillings were replaced. This was the first sign of improvement. -Weight loss -- I lost nearly 11 pounds from 135 to 124 despite eating large amounts of healthy, nutritious foods. Rash -- Reddish seborrhea-type [red, scaly and crusty] rashes on sides of nose and on scalp.

Incidentally, my symptoms began three days after running in the San Francisco Marathon in 1983. Perhaps the stress of the 26.2 mile run started the ball rolling. Interestingly, these symptoms were not contagious. My girlfriend from June 1983 to June of 1984 never once had any of these symptoms and really couldn't identify with what I was telling her . . .

All I can say is that gradually, over the course of one year after my fillings were replaced, I am about 95% cured.

I would like to recommend the following strategies which I feel quite literally saved my life:

1. REMOVAL OF FILLINGS [MERCURY FILLINGS] and replacement with non-metal ones -- they match the color of the teeth and are cosmetically more attractive!

2. Maintenance of a LOW-BLOOD-SUGAR DIET . . .

This way of eating has worked wonders for me! Carlton Fredricks and others write good books on the subject of low blood sugar.

3. REDUCTION OF ENDURANCE-TYPE EXERCISES & HIGH-STRESS LIFESTYLE

A) get plenty of sleep!

B) try to slow down your pace of living!

C) do things you really enjoy!

I can attest to these strategies because they really work. At present, I am a SPECIAL ED teacher with the New York City Board of Education and am the president of . . . a company which I brainstormed while recuperating from my "unknown" illness. Additionally, I have regained my strength to such a degree that I will be competing in [the] August SWIM-BIKE-RUN TRIATHLON CHAMPIONSHIPS in NEW YORK CITY (1 mile swim - 30 mile bike - 6.2 mile run non-stop).

I hope I have been of help to someone who is going through these symptoms . . . Thank you for helping me solve a two-and-one-half-year-long mystery!

Andrew J. Edelman
New York

Next is a letter from one of my patients who suffered from Chronic Fatigue Syndrome. Even though I knew by several past experiences what good changes were possible once she became mercury-free, I did not tell them to her for I did not want to prejudice her in any way. Besides, I had no way of knowing what changes would occur because there are no tests for determining this. I also asked that she wait several months after the last amalgam removal to report how she was doing so that she would be able to judge the longer–term results, as well as the short-term ones. Her letter explains her story well.

25

Dr. Hardy,

It has been four months since you completed removal of my amalgam fillings, including two mercury "balls" in the root from two old root canals. I cannot tell you how much better I feel! It has made all the difference in the world to my health.

As you may recall, I am a bit of a health fanatic and have been most of my adult life. I have done various things through the years to improve the quality of my health, from vitamins to diet to holistic doctors to kinesiology, some with good results and some with no results. I do not think that good health is the result of one thing, but more a combination of several things, [including] your spiritual and mental outlook. But without reservation, I can say that the removal of my amalgams has had the greatest single impact on my health of all the things I have done . . . their removal has resulted in visible, dramatic improvements. I appreciate you, your staff, and the research you have done in this field. THANK YOU!!

Tommie Bennett
Florida

This letter from a young lady in California tells about her recovery from headaches, fatigue, weakness and depression (sounds a little like CFS). She was only 14 when she went from sickness to health. She wrote the following letter when she was 16:

Dear [Dr.] Hardy,

. . . Before having all [my] mercury [fillings] removed, I had bad headaches all the time. I was tired and weak also. I was very depressed and quiet. Since I have had [my] mercury [fillings] removed, I don't have problems with any of the above. My family and friends say that I am more outgoing since my mercury has been removed . . .

Annamarie Anthony
California

Annamarie had her mercury amalgams replaced in 1985. She wrote to me in 1986. I called her in 1994 to follow up on her condition. We had a good talk and she sent the following letter:

Dr. Hardy,

. . . As you know, I had my mercury fillings removed in 1985 as I was having a lot of difficulties which my family thought were related to the fillings. I was previously easily fatigued and often ill. I have been doing well. I recently completed my master's degree and received my certification as a rehabilitation counselor. I currently work for the state of California as a [rehabilitation] counselor. I will continue my education to receive my PhD in the near future. I feel that I would not have had the energy to complete my graduate degree, especially while working full time, without having had these fillings removed and replaced . . . I . . . hope that my previous experience with mercury fillings will help others with the same symptoms.

Annamarie Anthony, M.A., C.R.C.
California

The next letter was written by a chiropractic physician who had gouty pains, chronic canker sores and short-term memory loss. He decided to replace his mercury amalgams to see if it would help.

Dear Dr. Hardy,

. . . After having been on an extensive health program for seven years, most of my physical problems had cleared beautifully. A canker sore problem which I had had since early childhood still remained, however. In the six-month period prior to my initiation of amalgam removal, I began experiencing a progressively worsening problem with short-term memory loss and severe shoulder and toe pain (much like gout). All of these were, in fact, threatening my career as a Doctor of Chiropractic.

After the removal of the amalgam fillings, there was an immediate change in all of these symptoms. Over a period of time, all symptoms have completely vanished except for an occasional canker sore. Even these are less frequent and less intense.

I thank you for your excellent care and for your pioneering work in this area of endeavor.

Philip Haselden, Jr., D.C.
Florida

There are currently no tests to determine if mercury causes arthritis or how much removing a chronic source of mercury from the body could help arthritis. It is common knowledge, however, that exposure to mercury can cause the identical joint pain found in arthritis (see rheumatoid arthritis, page 110). I am convinced that chronic exposure to mercury from amalgams is a contributing factor in some forms of arthritis.

I have had many rheumatoid arthritis (RA)-suffering patients find relief from simply removing amalgams and replacing them with composites. Some people get 10% better, others get 100% better. It seems to depend on their overall health, age, eating habits and the length of time they have had RA. In any case, who would want to be exposed to mercury, an element known to cause joint pain, especially if they were suffering from arthritis, a disease of unknown origins?

Based on my clinical experience and that of other mercury-free dentists, I am confident that at least partial recovery is possible in some diagnosed cases of arthritis. I do not promise patients any specific results. But I can say in general that previous mercury removal in arthritis patients has been quite successful in relieving joint pain (see Dr. Hardy's Arthritis Theory, page 111)

On page 111 is a letter from one of my patients diagnosed with RA. She found substantial relief when she replaced her mercury-containing fillings with composites. Her medical doctor wrote that her arthritis was in remission. It is important to note that RA is considered to be a chronic degenerative condition that has no cure. For a medical doctor to state that his patient's RA is in remission is extraordinary. Was it mercury poisoning from dental amalgam fillings that caused her RA?

Though dentists enjoy high patient respect and confidence, as well as good hours, it is common knowledge we have the highest rate of suicide of any profession. I believe it is a direct result of daily exposure to mercury vapor in the dental office. I believe dentists and dental assistants are harming themselves by working with amalgam.

The next letter is from a dental assistant in New Jersey. Dental assistants routinely prepare amalgam fillings for the dentist and, as a result, are exposed to mercury vapor daily. Studies in Denmark and Poland showed increased rates of spontaneous abortion in a group of dental assistants working with mercury.[19,20] The vast majority of dental assistants in the U.S. are women.

Dear Dr. Hardy,

My name is Colleen McBride. I am 20 years old . . . You have treated my dad and my brother, Richard C. McBride and Dr. Richard

29

Chapter 2

W. McBride. When my dad first went to you, he had headaches at least three times a week. He had them for years. The day you finished removing his amalgams, he felt as though a shade was lifted. That same night, he played racquetball and went swimming. He hasn't had a severe headache since. Maybe a dull ache once in a while, but nothing like before.

My brother was constantly chronically fatigued before you removed his amalgams. Now, he too is 100% better. He felt the same as my dad, as though a shade had been lifted off . . .

I truly believe that placing silver fillings in people's mouths is slowly killing the American population . . .

I started to work for an endodontist [root canal specialist]. I was his dental assistant. I loved the work I did. I worked three days a week. I guess it wasn't even quite a year that I started to notice a drastic change in my body. I was chronically fatigued all the time. I was starting to lose my memory . . . crying spells . . . crying constantly over nothing . . . major trouble making decisions. I actually felt like I was going crazy.

Before I worked as a dental assistant, I wanted to do everything. I was always active in snow skiing, weight-lifting and aerobics . . . a very active person. During the time I was sick, my body was constantly tight, I couldn't relax. I would get the shakes very bad . . . chest pains and constant headaches. I don't think it was so much the amalgams in my mouth, but being exposed to mercury vapor. As the doctor would drill out the silver [amalgam] to perform a root canal, I would be standing over the patient . . . inhaling.

Dr. Hardy, I would wake up in the morning and I was so scared of everything . . . right away I would cry . . . I would hardly sleep . . . getting scared of the dark. I would wake up . . . eat a little breakfast, stay in bed all day and night and cry and stare at the television. I was even losing track of time . . . I didn't want to see my friends or do anything, but hide from the world . . . I had no interest in life . . . I remember my mother hugging me and I said to her, "Mom, I just want to crawl under a rock and die!"

Just recently, [my dentist] took out my last [amalgam] . . . As the days went by, I started to feel better . . . I noticed I didn't feel like crying, I actually wanted to eat food. I wasn't better right away. It took about three weeks . . . My heart didn't ache anymore, my headaches stopped . . . my hearing was better, my sight was better and my sense of smell and taste was different also. I felt like I was more alert.

I remember sitting out on my back porch, taking in all the nature that was out there. I felt so good. I was enjoying life again. Since I am away from the dental office (I had to quit), and my [mercury] fillings are out, I'm not mean and miserable anymore. I [am] much happier and I don't see things negative[ly].

I owe everything to my family and to you Dr. Hardy, for doing all that research and believing in yourself . . . what you are doing is really helping people, it really is, look at me, I'm living proof!! I'm a totally different person.

Thank you so much.

Colleen McBride
New Jersey

I have been seeing more people with newly recognized problems called "environmental" illness. They can be characterized by a sensitivity to preservatives, food coloring, food flavoring, food additives, dyes, perfumes, certain types of air pollution, organic solvents found in paints, adhesives, building materials, cleaners, electromagnetic radiation and pesticides. Exposure to one chemical may trigger reactions to others. For some chemically sensitive individuals, mercury exposure may be the drop of water that spills the cup. It may be the one chronic exposure that makes all the other sensitivities worse. The next letter is from one of my most chemically sensitive patients.

Dear Dr. Hardy and staff:

. . . Removal of the mercury amalgams has been quite beneficial to me. It has generally made me feel better as well as increased my stamina. But one of the most noticeable improvements has been [in] my thinking processes.

Since my health problems are quite bad, this improvement was very much appreciated. I'm sure as time progresses and the mercury continues to be detoxed from my body, I'll have more areas of improvement, one of which I hope is the lessening of my chemical sensitivities. In my quest to regain my health, the removal of the mercury amalgam fillings has been the most beneficial treatment I have undergone, and I have undergone many.

Again, thank you for all your help and patience.

Cathy A. Altig
Florida

Those who are continually around us, such as family members, often see who we are better than we do. Likewise, we often see who they are better than they do.

Long-term low-level mercury exposure may be changing the personality of people to whom you are closest. The psychological symptoms of chronic mercury toxicity often creep up slowly (see "The Mad Hatters," page 131). And because there are a number of causes for personality changes, mercury poisoning may be overlooked.

The next letter is from a lady who, along with her husband, chose to have all of her mercury removed. I enjoy her description of how her husband has changed.

Dear Dr. Hardy,

The day following the removal of the last bit of mercury from my teeth, I realized my head felt pounds lighter (at least this is the way it felt). It was hard to believe that mercury caused such heaviness. My health has been decidedly better, and I'm able to maintain a cheerful attitude almost constantly. Last, but by no means least, my teeth no longer ache.

And as far as my appearance is concerned, my teeth look beautifully normal. When I smile, I no longer look like what I call a "metal-mouth."

My husband, Paul, is like a new person since he had all the mercury removed from his teeth. His health too, is much improved. However, the greatest improvement is in the fact that he is not as irritable as he used to be. He doesn't detect this change, but I can assure you, there is a definite difference.

Thank you for all the work you did on both of us. We are deeply and sincerely grateful.

Jeanne Hupper
Florida

Within my own family, my mother-in-law noticed a change in her husband after his mercury removal and periodontal cleanings.

My father-in-law had not seen a dentist in about 18 years when he came to me. We removed his mercury fillings and began a series of deep cleanings. My mother-in-law noticed a change in his personality immediately. She said he was more calm, patient and articulate. Interestingly, he hasn't noticed the change himself, but she would be the one to notice, since she interacts with him more than anyone else.

C h a p t e r   2

The next letter is written by a lady from Pennsylvania. It describes what she and her family went through on the road to recovery. I find interesting her humor, detail, and astute observations on the attitudes sometimes found among health care professionals.

Dear Dr. Hardy,

. . . I am a Caucasian female
Born October 31, 1930
5' 1 1/2" small frame, normal weight 110
4th of eight siblings (runt of the litter)
For the purposes of accuracy, I will try to get a copy of my records from my former dentist, but he may not be speaking to me. After he sent me a brochure from the American Dental Association stating that only 1% of the population is affected by mercury in fillings . . . [1% of the estimated people with amalgams are one million people] I returned a few selected articles for his enlightenment so that he could become aware and stop using amalgams (how naive!!) . . . oh, well . . .

Suffice it to say that I had a LOT of cavities in my teeth; all being filled with amalgam.

Age 13 — [I] could hear Dad's outgoing radio transmission when I was near the radiator, two floors up. No one else could. Dad didn't believe me until we both wrote down what he said.

Age 15 — [I] lost my first molar . . . it had a filling in it, but the pain was awful.

[My] allergies began in earnest. [I had my] first asthmatic attack . . . although I do not consider myself a true asthmatic since I am symptom-free between attacks . . . and GI upsets began about this time.

Age 19 — [I] noticed twitching of [my] eyelids. [I] needed to wear plain, but tinted eyeglasses, since my eyes were light sensitive. [Before losing my] upper molar, [the] pain was extreme. Nursing school would not give me two days off to go home to the dentist and sent me to [a dentist. He pulled it and found] nothing wrong with the tooth. [I was] also bothered with loss of concentration, swelling of joints, mainly hands and knees [and] muscular aches and pains. [I] gave up nursing although I had wanted to be a nurse all my life. I still do. How could I hope to help anyone else when I felt so bad myself?

Age 35 — [I] married [and began seeing a] new dentist. He replaced all the old fillings with new amalgams. [He] said they had rotted underneath because I didn't go to the dentist ! ! !

Age 39 — I will never forget the day I got home from the dentist. As the novacaine wore off, the pain in my face became excruciating . . . like a branding iron on the nerve. I thought that the needle had hit the nerve and called the dentist for advice. Would you believe the "Take-two-aspirin-and-go-to-bed-for-a-nap-what-you-describe-is-impossible" routine ? ? ? Alone in a big house with three babies ? ? ? Take a nap ? ? ? By the time I fed them all lunch and put them down for their nap, I could hardly see, the pain was so bad. But I did take two aspirin and laid down with a prayer that my angel would wake me if any of the children needed attention . . .

Anyway, I went back to the dentist who could find nothing wrong and sent me to the doctor. The doctor said there was no facial neuralgia [severe, sharp pain along the path of a nerve] and returned me to the dentist. After a couple of rounds of this, the dentist had the audacity to suggest that maybe I was one of "those ladies" who are unhappy at home and had a crush on the dentist! I can't believe that I let my husband talk me into continuing with this dentist. That's how far off my reasoning was becoming.

The years up to [age 45] are a . . . progression of symptoms. Some that I had became more pronounced and new ones came along. By this time, the dentist was putting in gold caps . . . over the amalgams.

"Gold in contact with amalgam constitutes short-circuited, permanent galvanic cells where the electrolytes are constantly renewed.

"The principles of galvanic corrosion are simple: when two dissimilar metals are in contact with an electrolyte, the less noble one [amalgam] is attacked and the more noble one [gold] is protected . . . many dentists prefer not to use silver amalgams adjacent to gold fillings because slight electrolytic action can promote toothache." (Encyclopedia Britannica Vol.8, page 239, 1965 edition) Now they tell me!

The most distressing to me were my mood swings. I was always kind of a naive dreamer who looked on the sunny side, I never had any problems, only opportunity to make things better. Now I found myself depressed, and really for no good reason. There was no financial worry . . . I had beautiful, healthy children, a wonderful husband who had no horrible vices and was always gentle. Why did I have these crying jags? Why was I anxious and afraid? Irish as I am? [I], who used to double-dare anyone? I was devastated with my feeling of confusion and inability to cope. Me, the great organizer! Me, the one who was always in control!

I can remember locking myself in the bathroom and splashing cold water on my face so that I would be able to go out and deal with the children. Where the unwarranted anger came from, I don't know. I wouldn't get in the car and drive alone to a place where I had never been for fear of getting lost. Also, I recall times (many times) looking at a person and saying "Uh-huh" [at] the proper intervals and when the conversation ended, would wonder what was said . . .

Age 45 — [I had a] complete hysterectomy. Non-cancerous.

Age 46 — [I had an] over-active thyroid, [was] tested for a year, given therapeutic dose of radioactive iodine, [it] returned to normal [without] medication.

Physical symptoms still persist[ed], but after so many years, they [became] just a part of my life. The persistent headache which [did] not respond to aspirin, the feeling of pressure over the right ear . . . like a hairband on too tight[ly], the ache in the right cheek bone (same side as the "neuralgia"), and most annoying [was] the tingling of the last three fingers of my right hand. If I kept using [my right hand], it would become numb with complete loss of feeling. [I] consulted the doctor because I was tired all day long, but just lay awake all night. [I was] not worrying or tossing and turning, just awake, like a zombie. The doctor was amused by my vagueness, but then he always was. On the other hand, my dentist could never understand why I always had a metal taste in my mouth [or] why my gums kept receding (which he treated by putting in more amalgam which turned black within a week.)

Age 54 — By this time, my alertness was reduced to a glassy-eyed stare. With much effort, I managed to wander through a day of not really doing anything . . . just getting up and getting to bed. I didn't really care. I was less than 96 pounds and looked like something the cat dragged in. The itching deep inside my ears was driving me nuts. It would wake me up at night.

In October 1985, [a dentist] began removing the amalgams from my mouth. After each visit, I felt ill for about three days. When he got around to the lower right jaw, while he was drilling, I felt the same awful itch inside my ear!

Age 56 — [In] May 1986, [my nutritionist] cannot believe how well I am . . . after just six months. NO depression ! ! ! NO muscular aches or pain. NO joint swelling. NO constant headache. NO "sinus trouble." NO metal taste. If I want to travel, I just get in the car and go. If the map gets me lost, I can stop and ask. What freedom!! My teeth are still crooked, but [I] no longer [have] the unsightly black [fillings] . . . I CAN COPE ! ! !

My feeling about the whole experience? Well, I thank God that I did finally find out what was wrong with me and was able to get it corrected.

I am sad for what my life could have been had I not been poisoned with mercury by the very people to whom I had entrusted my health.

But most of all, I am angry with the informed professionals who continue to poison children by putting mercury in their teeth. We are all made of the same stuff. If mercury poisoned me this much, even the person at the other end of the scale is poisoned somewhat. And one never knows which end of the scale he is on until it is too late. With other materials available, why do we take chances?

. . . The only thing to do is to inform the public.

Sometimes when I think over how I used to feel . . . that off-the-wall rage . . . I wonder how many people in our jails have amalgams in their teeth? . . .

Back in October [1985], when I started with [my nutritionist] and [dentist], I challenged my family . . . If they saw me get well, they would have their teeth made amalgam-free.

Although they too were ill for a few days following each visit, I am happy to say that all are feeling better. My daughter has not had a migraine headache since her amalgams were removed . . . She had been having them with increasing frequency and severity. My youngest son remarked that he feels more alert and sleeps better at night and no longer has a vague headache. His allergies are also improving.

Thank you for the opportunity to "join the fight!"

Joan D.
Pennsylvania

In the face of health challenges, many of us would just say, "I'm getting older" and "My body's falling apart". But I believe our bodies are made better than that. I see health as a picture containing many elements.

One is do no harm. The first step in achieving optimum health is to remove any substances from your life that are harmful. Mercury from amalgam is harmful in my opinion and should not be in any teeth.

I wish to address the part in Joan's letter where she felt badly after each amalgam removal visit. My partner also had showed no signs of mercury poisoning before her amalgam removal, but felt flu-like symptoms for several hours after each removal visit. This is not uncommon, even with extra precautions taken. Why? As the amalgams are being drilled out, a temporarily large concentration of mercury vapor exists in the mouth and in the air near the mouth, and the patient may breathe some.

But the good news is, once the fillings are out, exposure to their mercury vapor ceases. Certain vitamins and minerals help detoxify the body after amalgam removal. (They are covered on page 230.)

The only real change in dentistry will come from people who tell their dentist that they want change. I tried for years after dental school to make a difference by writing to the FDA, hundreds of congressmen and senators and dozens of organizations set up to help people with MS, arthritis, cancer, Lupus and other diseases. Some letters were unanswered, others sent form-letter replies and others answered with, "There is no scientific evidence of any connection between our disease and mercury exposure from dental fillings." I could get no real interest generated. So I realized I had to go straight to the public.

This book is written to you and for you. Take whatever information that is useful to you and pass along anything others may be able to use. In this way, public pressure to change amalgam use will grow. Thank you for your support in what I feel is a very important health issue.

Maybe one of these letters has struck a chord of harmony within you. Maybe you have a story to tell that you want others to read. Send it to me in care of Gabriel Rose Press; I will be honored and happy to read it and possibly include it in future editions.

Why was amalgam invented?

Why, if mercury is so poisonous, was amalgam ever invented or used in the first place? What's the story? The next chapter answers this question and raises more.

3

Chapter 3: Twinbirth: Amalgam and the ADA

hiding

truth

Twinbirth: Amalgam and the ADA

What is the American Dental Association?

The American Dental Association (ADA) is a non-governmental professional membership organization. It disseminates information to its members and the public, holds conventions, accepts and certifies dental products and devices and lobbies local, state and federal government officials in order to promote its specific positions.

The ADA has no legal authority. It makes no laws, enforces no laws, grants no licenses and cannot revoke any licenses. However, nearly all the legal bodies governing dental laws and licenses, from the local to the state to the federal levels are staffed by ADA members. Most local and state review or grievance boards are staffed with ADA members. In addition, most all the dentists teaching in dental schools across our country are ADA members. So the ADA has insiders everywhere in the system. Its interests are very well protected indeed.

Many states, including my own, Florida, require that a dentist who wants to become a member of a local or state dental organization must also become a member of the ADA. I cannot be a member of these societies because I choose not to be a member of the ADA. I smell monopoly and it's no game!

Your dentist may not know there is a problem with mercury amalgam because the ADA still claims there are no real problems with it and most dentists want to believe their own national membership organization. Even the ADA's own publications have contained reports enumerating amalgam's drawbacks, yet it remains supportive of mercury in teeth. The ADA finds no problem in using mercury as a chewing surface, so it attempts to paint mercury-free dentists as unethical. Ironically, while extolling the safety of mercury amalgam to the public, the ADA has taken the time to issue three pages of detailed mercury hygiene recommendations for the safety of all dentists and dental personnel.

This chapter examines some of the ADA's mercury hygiene recommendations. They clearly indicate the ADA is aware of at least some of the hazards of mercury.

This chapter also explores a brief history of mercury, the birth of amalgam and the founding of the ADA. I shall explain why amalgam became so popular and the reasons why the ADA continues to support mercury, a poison more dangerous than lead or arsenic.

Mercury, a poison then, a poison now

The best test for what is truth is to see how it remains true throughout time. Much wisdom which we hold dear today came from Greek and Roman philosophers and scientists who knew almost 2,000 years ago of mercury's dangerous properties. In the first century A.D., the Roman naturalist Pliny the Elder wrote in his Naturalis Historiae Libri, that mercury was a poison and had no business being used in medicine.[21,22]

The alchemists, practitioners of chemistry, loved mercury in the Dark and Middle Ages. It was a time filled with superstition and fear. They believed mercury could magically transmute base metals into gold. Hoping to strike the perfect combination that would create gold from another metal, they used it often in their work. They also thought it had magical healing properties, so many love potions and remedies for diseases of the time contained mercury.[23]

At first blush, the use of mercury in dentistry defies rational explanation when one realizes that five hundred years ago, mercury's detrimental effects on human teeth and gums were already known. Harmful effects including loosening of the teeth and bleeding gums were described by Alessandro Benedetti of Verona (1460-1525), one of the more important authors of the 15th century.[24]

First mercury fillings, 1601

The earliest written record of mercury being tried in a dental filling was in 1601. A German named Tobias Dorn Kreilius described the process as dissolving copper sulfide with strong acids, adding mercury, bringing the mixture to a boil and pouring it directly in the tooth cavity.[25] OUCH! I'd rather give my thumbnail a sharp whack with a hammer! Somehow this technique was not met with great enthusiasm by the public.

George Washington's death, 1799

The circumstances of George Washington's death are nothing less than barbaric by today's standards. Mercury is involved in his last days. In December 1799, Washington, feeling a cold come on, summoned his doctor. His doctor bled him several times, gave him a dose of mercury, bled him again and gave him a second dose of mercury. President Washington died the next day.[26] Of what then did the loved and honored Father of our Country die? Was it from his cold, the bleedings, or the mercury?

Hot fillings

In France they weren't doing much better for the poor, suffering patient. Those calling themselves dentists used a filling containing bismuth, tin and lead. It was also poured, boiling, into the screaming patient's teeth. They called this traumatic material D'Arcet's Mineral Cement.[27] One can only imagine the intensity of pain one must have been suffering before visiting the dentist in order to tolerate this kind of tortuous relief.

Finally, a Frenchman named Louis Regnart took pity on the patient and attempted to find an alternative to this dental torture. He increased the mercury concentration in the D'Arcet's Mineral Cement. This significantly lowered the temperature of the amalgam being placed in the cavity. Regnart's achievement bestowed upon him the title "Father of Amalgam."

Around the time Regnart was lowering the temperature of amalgam, the first experiment to demonstrate the toxic effects of mercury on unborn insects was done. Another Frenchman, Gaspard, exposed one group of fly eggs to mercury vapor while protecting another group from it. Both sets of eggs were kept at acceptable temperature and humidity levels. Not a single egg hatched in the

45

mercury-exposed group. Hundreds of eggs hatched in the non-exposed group.

Room-temperature fillings, 1826

In 1826, just six years after Gaspard's experiment, another Frenchman, M. Traveau, mixed pure silver powder with mercury and called it pate' d'argent (silver paste). This mixture could be placed in a tooth cavity at room temperature. The one drawback his amalgam had was that it expanded uncontrollably after being placed in the tooth. This ultimately caused the patient's tooth to split like a log under an axe.[28] And remember, there was no such thing as novacaine or nitrous oxide to lessen the pain in those days.

A lot was happening in France, but in the U.S., dentistry was taking shape as a separate profession from medicine.

Dentistry split off as a profession separate from medicine from 1780 to 1800 in the United States.

There were two types of "dentists" at this time. There were medical doctors trained to practice both medicine and dentistry, called medical-dentists. Then there were:

"those who were merely craftsmen and engaged in some other trade, such as barbering, carving of wood, ivory and metals . . . among them were the itinerant tooth pullers."[29]

They were called the craftsmen-dentists.

Before 1840, there were no dental schools, no dental licensing, no national dental organizations and no dental board exams. Dentists were either self-taught by trial and error or were apprenticed under a practicing medical-dentist.

Today it is taken for granted that your dentist has graduated from an accredited dental school after receiving a college education. After graduating with a doctorate degree, the dentist must pass a rigorous national board exam and a state or regional board exam. Further, licensing is required by state or by region. In addition, states require continuing education as a requirement in licensing while in practice.

None of this was true in the 1830s when amalgam was introduced in the U.S. Anybody could be a dentist. All one had to do was to hang a shingle on the shack and POOF, instant dentist.

Anybody who so desired could set himself up in practice with no more requirements than the opening of a blacksmith shop. In fact, during early colonial days the blacksmith often used his tongs as forceps for tooth extraction.[30] A typical sign might have read:

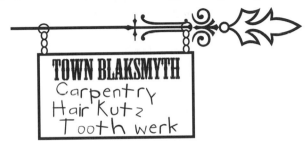

If one had a cavity in the 1830s, the dentist might use a file on the tooth as described in this excerpt from an 1845 dental textbook:

"The file, during the operation should be frequently dipped in water, so as to prevent it from becoming heated, or choaked between the teeth . . . The sensation produced by filing the teeth, is, to most persons, disagreeable and, to some, positively painful . . .[31]

There were no drills and no anesthesia.

Chapin Harris, an M.D. and dentist, was likely the most respected medical-dentist of the 1830s to the 1860s. He was the author of two of the first dental textbooks and co-founder of the world's first dental school. In one of his textbooks, he describes the quality of dentistry during the early 1800s:

"In 1830, the number of Dentists in the United States, according to the best information which the author has been able to obtain, was about three hundred, but of these, not more perhaps, than forty or fifty had attained too much knowledge in any of the departments of the art. The portals of the profession then, as now [1845], were open to the ignorant as well as the educated and in consequence of this, its members multiplied rapidly."[32]

This lack of checks and balances in the 1830s in the dental field left it wide open to swindlers and con artists. Prior to the introduction of amalgam, medical concerns were foremost in the minds of most dentists. Amalgam changed the focus of fillings from medicine to mechanics. Medical-dentists and craftsmen-dentists were now at odds. First, we will meet the most infamous con artists and swindlers in the history of dentistry.

Amalgam introduced by con men

The Crawcours brothers introduced the mercury amalgam filling first to England and then to the United States. They are the most notorious schemers in the history of dentistry. They knew enough about dentistry to predict large financial gain in using this new mercury filling. The huge profit they accumulated in Britain as a result of its advertisement and use was a confirmation.

With the introduction of the mercury filling, they knew that patients now had another choice with which to get a cavity fixed. Previously, the patient had two options. The first was extraction of the tooth with no anesthesia (in the 1830s, local anesthesia had not yet been invented.) The second was a long appointment in which hot gold would be hammered into the tooth. The new third choice was the Crawcours' "silver" filling which they claimed would fill the tooth cavity painlessly in minutes. It is clear why amalgam became the most widely used dental material in history. Effective advertising was the key in selling the mercury filling to the public.

Mercury amalgam was the first inexpensive, room-temperature filling material ever available. The dental consumer finally got an easy-to-take filling. In Europe, the Crawcours brothers called their filling MINERAL SUCCEDANEUM. They profited hugely, but they decided they could make even more by embellishing their advertising before exporting it to the United States. So they changed the name of their filling material to ROYAL MINERAL SUCCEDANEUM. The Crawcours brothers knew the public associated the term "royal mineral" with gold. They did not advertise the use of mercury in the filling even though it was the main ingredient. Effective advertising targeted the public's wants and outflanked the medical profession's opposition.

Today, effective advertising still cloaks the major ingredient in amalgam. By calling amalgam a "silver" filling, most dentists deceive the public about its composition. Even though mercury has always been the main ingredient, amalgam has never been called a mercury filling.

Instant wealth, lasting damage, 1833

Let's back up a bit to 1833 when the Crawcours brothers brought amalgam to New York in the midst of what was described as an advertising avalanche. Extensive flashy advertisements along with a sumptuous plush New York office gave them instant wealth and fame.[33]

Their ROYAL MINERAL SUCCEDANEUM sounded like gold but was inexpensive compared to the real gold being used by reputable dentists. They could charge less while profiting more. It was a slick operation. They removed good gold work and put their own cheap amalgams in its place. They packed amalgam between teeth that had no decay. They crammed amalgam over decay without it first being removed. And, to shape the filling, they had the patient bite down on a blob of amalgam, forcing the unsuspecting soul to swallow any excess mercury and silver.[34]

How could the patients know what was being done? There was no indication in the advertising that a poisonous ingredient, mercury, was being used. And, although their money may have been taken for worthless fillings, they had no pain during the procedure. Patients assumed that if the dental work was painless, it was good as well as safe.

The advent of mercury amalgam to the U.S. was noticed and opposed by the leading medical-dentists. Chapin Harris, in his text-book on dental surgery, wrote this about amalgam:

"The amalgam of mercury and silver, . . . is decidedly the most pernicious material that has ever been employed for filling teeth."[35]

Pernicious in Webster's unabridged dictionary means destructive; having the power of killing, destroying, ruining, or injuring; fatal; deadly or wicked; evil.

Dr. Harris and others knew that it was the mercury that was dangerous:

"Some have endeavored to obviate the objection to this amalgam by using silver perfectly purified, but it matters not how pure the silver may be, the material will be equally deleterious in its effects . . . It is the mercury that does the injury and it matters not therefore, how pure or what the other metal may be that is employed with it for the formation of the amalgam."[36]

One of his concerns centered around the widespread use of amalgam by uneducated and unskilled dentists. Another concern was about the misleading and dishonest advertising of amalgam:

"This article [amalgam] has been extensively used and highly puffed, by a certain class of practitioners, during the last five or six years, both in the United States and England, but it has had its day and I am happy to believe, that it is not at present employed by any scientific or respectable practitioner."[37]

Dr. Harris was right about amalgam not being used by any scientific or respectable practitioner of his day, but he was entirely wrong about amalgam already having its day. He would be disheartened and dismayed to know that 160 years later amalgam is still having its day.

The Amalgam War (1833-199?)

The bitter controversy between craftsmen-dentists and medical-dentists over mercury amalgams began what continues to be known as the Amalgam War.

"The amalgam war was the war between the craftsmen ideal of ease of manipulation and the medical ideal of the avoidance of danger of systemic mercurial poisoning."[38]

Mercury was clearly known to be poisonous to the medical-dentists of the 1830s.

Craftsmen-dentists were not concerned with the medical consequences of placing mercury into their clients' teeth. However, in their defense, I believe the craftsmen-dentists thought that amalgam was fine. Ignorance, not malice, was the root of their belief. Anatomy, chemistry, histology, pathology and physiology were considered irrelevant to the craftsmen. Their only concerns were that amalgam was easy to use, filled the hole and was profitable. Their patients were convinced that amalgams were good because they were inexpensive and filled the cavities in their teeth quickly with no pain, just as the Crawcours brothers had advertised.

Unfortunately, patients of today, just like yesterday, trust that their dentist is using the best materials. Few people, then or now, knew that mercury was and is, the major ingredient in their so-called "silver" fillings.

The medical-dentists believed that something had to be done. There seemed to be deteriorating concern and increasing ignorance for the patients' medical welfare as evidenced by the growing use of amalgam. So, the medical-dentists created the world's first dental school and the first national dental organization in order to raise the standards of dental education and care.

World's first dental school, 1840

Craftsmen-dentists strongly resisted the dental school's formation. They did not want to be forced to go to school to be dentists. The less-expensive trial-and-error training was preferred. They also believed that the school's medical-dentist teachers were using the dental students for selfish profit. The resistance by the craftsmen-dentists was substantial: 24 years after the first American dental school opened, only four dental schools existed.

The first dental school in the world, the Baltimore College of Dental Surgery, was chartered on February 1, 1840. The Board of the College of Dental Surgery was composed of nine physicians, five clergymen and, ironically, no dentists. The school's founders, Dr. Chapin A. Harris and Dr. Horace Hayden, considered two of the most respected pioneers of dental education, are credited as the driving forces behind dentistry's recognition as a separate and distinct specialty of the healing arts.

Originally, the school was to be a graduate program for medical schools. Dentistry was intended to be a specialty of medicine. It was only one session long and did not include any chemistry or pathology.[39,40]

In defining the school's purpose, Harris wrote:

"The object of this institution is, to give those who receive its instructions, a thorough Medico-dental education, so that when they enter upon the active duties of the profession, they may be enabled to practice it, not alone as a mere mechanical art, but upon sound scientific principles, as a regular branch of medicine. While the head is being educated in such branches of general medicine and Surgery, . . . the fingers of the Student, are, at the same time, regularly drilled every day in the various mechanical manipulations belonging to it . . . This fact, it is believed, will ever connect the destinies of the Institution with the welfare of the profession in this country.

"Nor will its salutary influence stop here. It will be felt in other countries and will be instrumental in elevating the standard of Dental qualifications everywhere." [41]

Later dudes!

The medical-dentists of New York decided it was important to have a dental society composed of reputable dentists to protect the public from charlatans such as the Crawcours brothers. So in 1834, they formed the first dental society in the United States. It was through the efforts of this society that the Crawcours brothers were actually run out of the country. [42]

Most dentists unqualified, 1842

According to Harris, there were about 1,400 dentists in the U.S. in 1842 and:

"Many, very many, of those engaged in the practice at present, possess but few and some none, of the necessary qualifications for it." [43]

Amalgam was apparently first used by the uneducated, unqualified dentists. As the numbers of mercury-using dentists grew, the medical-dentists realized that, in order to protect the public health, they had to take a stand.

Amalgam use declared malpractice in 1843

The state dental society in New York was a good start toward creating a conscience for the profession, but a national organization would be able to raise the standards of all dental care in the country. So, in 1840, a few months after the chartering of the Baltimore College of Dental Surgery, the world's first national dental organization, the American Society of Dental Surgeons (ASDS) was formed.

A resolution passed by the ASDS in 1843 stated that the use of amalgam was considered to be malpractice. Members pledged to not use mercury fillings and to oppose their use under any circumstances. Those members that refused to sign the pledge were expelled from the society.

The first and second casualties of the Amalgam War, 1856

The Amalgam War was escalating. Not all the ASDS members were happy about the ban against amalgam use. Some wanted to use amalgam to remain competitive. From the patient's point of view, the comparative ease and affordability of mercury fillings kept amalgams in high demand. More and more members of the ASDS chose to use amalgam rather than lose patients. As a consequence, the membership and influence of the ASDS began to dwindle.[44,45] In hopes of gaining more members, the ASDS decided to rescind its anti-amalgam resolution in 1850, but the lack of membership money caused the ASDS to eventually disband in 1856. [46]

So, the first casualty of the Amalgam War was individual medical ethics, cut down by business pressures to survive. The second casualty was the altruistic and honorable American Society of Dental Surgeons.

Prior to the demise of the ASDS, dentists using mercury were meeting and associating with one another. They knew they had a filling material the public wanted. After all, it was placed in the cavity at room temperature, not boiling hot like some fillings of the day. And amalgam was more profitable for the dentist and less expensive for the patient. Almost everyone could afford it and it made money for the dentist. The amalgam-using dentists wanted to form their own organization.

This led to the formation, in 1859, of the dental organization called the American Dental Association. (I like to call the ADA the Amalgam Dental Association.) According to an article written in *Dental Students' Magazine* of September 1943, the typical dentist in the ADA was no longer in sympathy with medicine. Members' interests and concerns rested with the mechanical, rather than medical aspects of dentistry. Because of this approach, the physicians of the day adopted a progressively disapproving attitude toward dentistry.

During this same time, dental schools dropped courses in physiology, pathology, materia medica (medical matters) and did no anatomy except head and neck. [47]

I don't know a single patient of mine whose head is not connected to his body. To drop such courses was an insult to the Hippocratic code of above all, DO NO HARM. It's as though the dental profession was saying teeth are separate from the body and have no influence over and are not affected by, what occurs elsewhere in the body. Great philosophers have always known that we are whole beings: physical, emotional and spiritual.

A tale of two dentists, 1860

Let's look at two dentists who could have lived during the time when amalgam was introduced to the U.S., Drs. Henry Truman and Wayne Payne. These fictitious dentists were on opposite sides of the Amalgam War.

Chapter 3

Truman was a physician who studied under the leading dentist of his day and became a fine medical-dentist. Truman had the medical education to know that mercury was a known poison and, therefore, must not be used in dental fillings.

Wayne Payne was a skilled ivory carver, blacksmith, carpenter and barber. Many of his clients who came for a shave wanted a tooth filled or pulled as well. He was more than happy to oblige, wielding the same tongs he used to pull nails from horses' hooves. When he began to use amalgam, he noticed he could fill some teeth he would have normally extracted. Word got around and he became busy filling teeth with amalgam. Payne found that fillings were quite profitable, so he decided to become a dentist.

To do that, all he had to do was tell people he was a dentist. Payne did not have to take any schooling, exams, or apprenticeships. He was a crafstman-dentist. It did not matter that he had no medical background and was unaware mercury was so poisonous. He only knew that for the first time, he had a filling material that could fill teeth quickly and profitably.

There was no anesthesia for him to use. Before mercury amalgams were available, the patient's choice was limited to having the decayed tooth extracted, having a boiling lead filling or having an expensive hot gold filling hammered into the tooth: all very painful. Payne did not know how to use gold and the new mercury fillings were affordable to nearly everyone. He saw a big future ahead as a mercury-using dentist. Patients filled up his barn wanting the new type of filling.

Even some patients of Truman, the physician-dentist down the street, began coming to Payne because they heard how cheap and painless his fillings were. Truman was sad that these patients did not know what was being put in their mouths. Amalgams were being called "silver" fillings, not "mercury" fillings. And Payne only cared that amalgam filled the cavity, not that mercury was harmful. Eventually, Truman had almost no dental patients because he did not use mercury. It was against his medical judgment to use mercury, so he quit dentistry and became a writer rather than debase his ethical values.

Payne's friends saw him making lots of money as a dentist, so, an increasing number of his craftsmen buddies became dentists. There was just one problem tarnishing their use of the new mercury filling: The first and quite well-respected national dental society in America, the American Society of Dental Surgeons (ASDS). It had declared the use of mercury amalgam malpractice saying that amalgam contained the poison mercury.

Certainly, Payne was distressed when his patients questioned his use of mercury. Payne just told them there was nothing to the claims that mercury amalgams cause any medical problems. Even though he was not qualified to give this answer, he knew that most people wanted amalgam and that the mercury filling could make him a wealthy man. So he chose to ignore the warnings about mercury. Most patients believed his unqualified reassurances and he did not see any harm in its use.

For more prestige, Payne wanted to join the ASDS but couldn't because he used mercury. Many of his fellow mercury-dentists also wanted to become members of a dental organization and so, in 1859, they decided to form their own organization.

They called it the American Dental Association. The use of mercury was just fine with the ADA. Membership numbers grew quickly and the ADA did not mourn the demise of the American Society of Dental Surgeons in 1856.

Payne made lots of money. He ate and drank too much and died at an early age, of suicide. Truman became the owner of a successful publishing company, had two children and co-authored 15 books with his wife of 50 years. He died a happy man.

By 1884 there were 22 dental schools in the United States, most of them privately owned. But the medical side of dentistry was regressing instead of progressing.

Says one author on this era:

"The atmosphere at most private dental colleges was more nearly that prevailing in trade schools and this attitude naturally permeated to the student body, who gave but scant attention to any subject excepting those pertaining to the technical side of dentistry. Knowledge of anatomy, chemistry or histology was considered useless and a sheer waste of time."[48]

It was not until 1917 that even a high-school diploma was needed to enter dental school.[49]

It is amazing that it has only been in my grandmother's lifetime that dental education realized the indispensable value of medical training. Yet here we are, almost in the 21st century, still using 19th century amalgams.

For dentistry to step out of the 1830s and fully acknowledge its responsibility as a healing art, the use of mercury must again be declared malpractice, as it was over 150 years ago.

Rock and roll and the ADA

The ADA has been rocking and rolling since it first began in 1859. No other dental association in the world has had such a long history or so great an influence over its profession.

The ADA may owe all that it has become to the use of mercury-amalgam. Without mercury-amalgam, the ADA may never have been founded. Amalgam has allowed the ADA to grow and prosper. Amalgam has allowed the ADA to rock and roll over any competition. But now the ADA has rocked and rolled itself into a corner by stubbornly refusing to admit that good old mercury-amalgam may be causing patients harm. The problems resulting from amalgam use are heavily testing the ADA's credibility and moral character.

For instance, in 1990, "60 Minutes" newsmagazine did a damaging expose' on amalgam. Many patients began asking new questions about it. Never before did dentists have to answer so many questions on mercury. They were so overwhelmed that the ADA printed material for them to simply hand out to any patients with questions on amalgam. It was all the information dentists needed to answer questions on amalgam, according to the ADA. Some dentists were outraged that they should be told what to say to their patients by their dental organization, but most dentists bought the ADA line as truth. Besides, it was an easy way to placate the patients with the difficult questions. (More about the "60-Minutes" controversy later this chapter.)

Another sign that the amalgam issue is hurting the ADA is that the association has been losing members to other dental organizations.

Several of these organizations oppose the use of biologically incompatible dental materials, including mercury-amalgam. (I personally discontinued my membership in the ADA, because it continues to stonewall the evidence against amalgam. As always, the ADA says more research is needed.)

Because of the amalgam controversy, you could say that the ADA is now singing the blues: the amalgam blues. Worldwide, more and more dentists, physicians, health care professionals and patients are concluding that dental amalgams are dangerous and should be banned. The band is playing louder and louder and the ADA can't help but hear the music. Soon, the very existence of the ADA may be in jeopardy if it stubbornly holds to its mercury-amalgam position.

Ridicule and intimidation

The ADA has managed to obscure the mercury issue for 160 years. It has even broadened its power and influence through justifying amalgam use. A look at how the ADA has handled the amalgam war in the past 15 years demonstrates how a powerful organization can ridicule and intimidate those with opposing views. Such a strong association can fund studies and manipulate statistics in order to fit its hypothesis that no health risks exist from dental amalgam. Because of mounting scientific evidence and media attention against mercury in fillings, the ADA is becoming more frantic and harsh. Read on to understand some of the ploys used by the ADA.

ADA changes stand on mercury vapor from amalgam, 1981

Until the early 1980s, the ADA steadfastly claimed that mercury vapor did not escape from amalgams. In order to lend credence to its position, it quoted outdated research done in the mid-1950s. Then, in the early 1980s, the ADA reversed its stand by admitting that mercury vapor does escape from amalgam.

A group from the University of Iowa, headed by Dr. Carl W. Svare, showed conclusively that mercury vapor does escape from amalgam fillings in patients' mouths. In that study, patients with and without amalgams were measured for mercury vapor in exhaled breath. Those with amalgams showed a 15.6-fold increase in the amount of mercury vapor after chewing gum for only ten minutes. Those without amalgams showed no change.[50,51]

Common sense says, and research confirms, that mercury is constantly released from amalgam. Amalgam has been known to break, crack, wear down and fall out. This could only happen if the filling was deteriorating. Since the major part of amalgam is mercury, the filling loses mercury as it deteriorates.

I'm sure the intelligent researchers at the ADA knew this also, even though they formerly claimed just the opposite.

ADA standard operating procedures, 1982

Smoke screens set up by the ADA to turn attention away from the real issue of amalgam hazards are part of its standard operating procedures. It creates paper tigers for the profession as well as the public to chase. One example was set up for the profession in 1982. The ADA created a urinary mercury testing service to monitor the mercury exposure of dentists and staff. It claimed that the service was also somehow supposed to educate the dentists and staff on the hazards of mercury exposure.

The reasons given to the profession in 1982 for urinary testing directly contradicted the ADA's position stated in 1971. Then, the ADA's Council on Dental Materials and Devices and the Council on Dental Research said:

"The mercury level in the urine, therefore, is not dependable for toxic determinations . . . because the urinary level drops with the onset of symptoms of mercurial poisoning, this test is not dependable to determine toxic reactions." [52]

It is clear that the ADA knew that urinary mercury levels were not dependable, but it set up the testing service anyway. The ADA wanted to look as though it was concerned and diligent about the mercury issue. Besides, it probably knew that very few dentists understood that urinary mercury levels are inaccurate to worthless for diagnosis of chronic mercury poisoning.

So-called "accurate" information from the ADA to the patients, 1984

Another example of the slick way in which the ADA has been confusing the issue of amalgam safety was illustrated in a 1984

61

brochure directed first to the dentist and then to the patient. The ADA presented the issue as one of amalgam safety instead of mercury hazards:

"To help you provide accurate information to your patients on this issue (amalgam safety), the ADA has prepared a fact sheet that appears below. We suggest that you cut it out and reproduce it for distribution for those patients who express concern.

"To the dental patient:

"Recent reports in the public media have raised questions as to the safety of dental amalgam. In order to provide you with accurate information on the use and safety of dental amalgam, the American Dental Association has prepared the following answers to the most commonly asked questions about dental amalgam.

"Which metals are used in dental amalgam?

"Silver, copper and tin are the metals commonly used in dental amalgam, sometimes in combination with zinc."[53]

The answer does not include mercury. This is an obvious and blatant lie designed specifically to confuse the consumer. Mercury is a metal and it is the major metallic component of dental amalgam.

Up to 70% of an amalgam is mercury. Hmmm . . . forget to mention this for a particular reason? Later the ADA "fact sheet" admits mercury is used, but says:

"When mercury is combined with the metals used in dental amalgam, its toxic properties are made harmless." [54]

That's like saying when lead is combined with paint, its toxic properties are made harmless. Or when lead is combined with the glaze on dinner plates, its toxic properties are made harmless. Neither is true.

When mercury is mixed with the other metals in dental amalgam, it constantly evaporates from the filling in the form of mercury vapor. There is no way to render mercury vapor's toxic properties harmless. Dr. Lars Friberg, considered to be the world's leading expert on mercury poisoning said that there is no safe level of mercury and that there is no proof of any safe level.[55] Mercury vapor is released 24 hours a day from every single amalgam. Does the ADA really believe that the mercury vapor from amalgams is different from all other mercury vapor? Of course not.

This ADA "fact sheet" was yet another smoke screen set up to cloud the amalgam issue a while longer. And they are still playing games with words while evading the real issues of your best health, my best health and the best health of our planet.

What bothers me even more than this propaganda, spoon fed from the ADA to its members, who turn around and feed it to the public, is the high probability that most dentists reading this "fact sheet" may believe it. How many dentists do their own research to see if what is being told to them is, in fact, truth? They may be too busy, too comfortable and don't wish to appear controversial. The ADA provides slick and seemingly respectable answers. Don't most dentists hand this material to their patients fully believing it? Courage and energy are needed to search for the truth beyond what we are told is true.

It is easier to remain complacent and accept the status quo than to question long-held views. There even exists a tendency to deny opposing points of view when they undermine traditionally held ones. But truth persists through such resistance. Truth seems to move through three stages. First, it is denied. Second, it is forcefully opposed. Third, it is accepted as fact.

ADA recommendations on mercury hygiene, 1984

The ADA recommendations on mercury hygiene covers three pages in the October 1984 issue of its *Journal of the American Dental Association* (JADA). There are no recommendations for composite --

the non-toxic filling alternative -- hygiene, because none are needed. There would be no need for this extensive safety section if mercury, a known toxin, was not used by the profession.

The vast majority of the 193,000 practicing dentists use mercury. About 140,000 of them are ADA members.[56] Here are just some of the ADA's recommendations to dentists who use mercury:

*Mercury Sensitivity or Allergy

"In extremely rare cases, individuals may develop a mercury sensitivity or an allergy may be activated by contact with mercury. This can involve patients or dental office personnel." [57]

In fact, there are no studies that support the ADA's claim that mercury sensitivity and allergy are extremely rare. No one really knows if sensitivity is rare or common. But the ADA prefers to use the word rare and modify it by the word extremely. I believe when more definitive research is done on mercury sensitivity and allergy, it will be concluded that they are both more common than rare.

*Specific symptoms

"Specific symptoms of mercury exposure can include: tremor observable in fine voluntary muscular movements such as handwriting . . . eventually progressing to convulsions; loss of appetite; nausea and diarrhea; depression, fatigue, increased irritability, or moodiness; pneumonitis; nephritis; nervous excitability; insomnia; headache; swollen glands and tongue; ulceration of oral mucosa; and dark pigmentation of marginal gingiva and loosening of teeth." [58]

Fine, voluntary muscular movements such as those found in the intricate work of dentistry can also be adversely affected by mercury, but the ADA chose to say "handwriting." Depression, irritability and moodiness are often found among dentists. And the highest rate of suicide has been found to be among dentists. I believe it is caused by their daily dose of mercury at the office.

*Sources of mercury exposure

No less than eleven sources of mercury exposure in the dental office are listed by the ADA in its 1984 recommendations. The doctor, staff and patients can be exposed from any or all of these:

1. mercury spills (mercury that is used in the making of amalgam, or, presumably, from a broken mercury thermometer)

2. leaky mercury dispensers (dispensers are used for making amalgam) .

3. leaky amalgam capsules (the small containers used for making amalgam are called capsules. The amalgam inside is called a "spill")

4. contaminated amalgam capsules (used for making amalgam)

5. wringing excess mercury from amalgam (during the making of amalgam)

6. vaporization of mercury from contaminated instruments in sterilizers (all instruments and drill bits that have touched amalgam and that have not been cleaned perfectly)

7. amalgam condensation: ultrasonic condensing increases mercury exposure over hand condensing (putting the amalgam into a tooth is called condensation)

8. scrap amalgam improperly stored (The amalgam left over after part of it is placed in a tooth as a filling is called scrap. Scrap amalgam should be stored away from any source of heat in a tightly closed container under a sulfur-containing liquid such as X-ray fixer solution containing sulfuric acid.)

By definition, then, amalgam in the mouth is improperly stored. The mouth is not cold nor is it a tightly closed container, nor is there a sulfur solution covering the amalgam[s].

9. organic mercurial disinfectants (I know of no dentist who uses such disinfectants, as they have not been shown to be effective. Two cases in point; the presumed antiseptics called Mercurochrome and Merthiolate, both containing mercurial disinfectants, have been removed from the market by the FDA due to lack of effectiveness)

10. removing old amalgam restorations (this happens anytime a filling is ground out for a new filling or ground down for a crown or a bridge, a common procedure)

11. contaminated amalgamators (the machine used to mix amalgam is called an amalgamator)[59]

Only source #10 above -- amalgam removal-related hazards -- exists with the exclusive use of the stronger, safer and more attractive composite resin fillings. Special precautions are taken by many mercury-free dentists to minimize the mercury exposure a patient may receive during amalgam removal. Items #1 - 9 and 11 would not apply in a mercury-free office. Therefore, 10 out of 11 sources do not exist in a mercury-free practice.

*The Mercury Work Area

The mercury work area is the room in which a patient sits while having amalgam placed. The center of the mercury work area is the patient's mouth. The ADA recommendations for the mercury work area include:

"The work area should be a well ventilated space with fresh air exchange and outside air exhaust." [60]

I happen to live and work in Florida. The idea of a fresh air exchange is a good one. However, the reality of keeping cool in 96 degree, 96% humidity heat is something else. There are many spring, summer and fall days where the air conditioner has a tough enough time keeping myself and my staff cool by recirculating indoor air. We must wear water resistant gowns over our scrubs, rubber gloves, glasses and a mask. It gets warm under there. Would you want an uncomfortable dentist and dental assistant working on a difficult procedure in your mouth?

"When mercury is handled and stored, impervious surfaces with restraining edges should be used." [61]

The mouth is neither an impervious surface, nor does it have restraining edges.

A 1971 ADA article reported that:

"The use of carpets in the office area for comfort and appearance has added an almost impossible obstacle to the recovery of mercury spills." [62]

In this article, carpet was not recommended in the dental operatory. The operatory is the room in which dental work is done.

"Design the dental office with seamless flooring that extends two inches up each wall." [63]

Two inches up the wall was fine in 1971, but in 1984 the ADA doubled that to four inches (10 cm):

"The use of a continuous seamless sheet for flooring carried up the walls for at least 10 cm offers easier and more efficient clean-up of mercury spills . . . The use of a carpeted floor . . . does not lend itself to complete decontamination except for removal of carpet." [64]

So, even though the ADA doubled the recommendation on wall coverage and noted that decontamination of carpets is impossible, it still hasn't pressed for legislation prohibiting carpet in the treatment areas. Why? My guess is that so many offices already are carpeted that the ADA would encounter vehement opposition from its members if it backed a mandate that required all carpeting be removed from dental operatories. Today, the expense of redoing the flooring takes priority over what is best for the health of everyone in the office, including the patient.

The ADA says that it only takes one mercury spill and the carpet cannot be cleaned. Only by removing the carpet will the spill be cleaned up. It is clear, then, that if a dentist works with mercury, he or she should not work over carpet. Someday, when the last amalgam is gone maybe dental offices could all have quiet, comfortable, attractive and safe carpeting again.

The ADA says it is not okay to leave mercury in the carpet, exposed to the office air, but it is okay to leave mercury amalgam in the mouth, exposed to the air drawn into the lungs all day and all night!

*Mercury and Amalgam Storage

The ADA said in 1984:

"Mercury should be stored in unbreakable, tightly sealed containers on stable surfaces and kept from any source of heat . . . A face mask should be used to avoid breathing amalgam dust." [65]

Body heat is a source of heat. Mercury should be kept from any source of heat. I agree.

Of course, the ADA fails to mention that a dust mask is worse than useless at keeping mercury vapor from getting into the lungs. A dust mask can trap small particles of amalgam on its surface and the heat from the dentist's breath can increase the mercury vapor released. Only a special mercury-absorbing mask will decrease the lungs' and airways' absorption of mercury vapor. Few, if any, mercury-using dentists use this type of mask.

Says the ADA:

"Ultrasonic condensors should not be used . . ." [66]

Ultrasonic condensors pack the filling in the tooth much faster than can be done by hand. They save time, make a better-packed filling and are probably sold by every dental supply company in the country. Does the ADA really think that dentists won't use them?

*Leftover amalgam scraps

"Each drain, vacuum, cuspidor or sink, into which scrap amalgam may enter, should be fitted with a filter, strainer or trap that will catch the particles." [67]

How much mercury goes down every dentist's drain? Where does the mercury go? See chapter 5, "Mercury on Earth," to understand the serious environmental consequences of dental mercury use. Remember that these are recommendations from an organization that denies there is any hazard in the use of amalgam.

"All amalgam scraps should be salvaged and stored in a tightly closed container. The scrap should be covered by a sulfide solution such as X-ray or photographic fixer solution . . . Contaminated disposable materials . . . should be placed in (plastic) bags and sealed before disposal . . . health or environmental agencies should be consulted for methods of disposing of the contaminated items." [68]

What makes amalgam scrap? If it is not in the tooth, it is called scrap. Environmental agencies must be contacted for proper disposal methods of that little piece of amalgam that didn't go in the tooth. If amalgam is unsafe to put in the trash can, is it safe in the mouths and bodies of an ADA estimate of 100 million Americans? [69]

*To vacuum or not to vacuum

"A household vacuum cleaner should not be used on mercury spills or on contaminated floors." [70]

All dental office cleaning services that clean amalgam-using offices should be properly warned of the possible hazards of vacuuming mercury-contaminated areas.

So, let's take a poll of 100 cleaning services all over the country that clean amalgam-using dental offices. Let's ask them if they have been informed of possible mercury exposure and how to deal with it. How many would you guess have been properly informed? How many services use an ordinary household vacuum? And does the cleaning service take the same vacuum to your tidy little abode less than ten minutes after cleaning two or more of the local mercury-using dental offices?

*Don't touch amalgam

"Direct contact or handling of mercury, amalgam or mercury-containing materials should be avoided." [71]

I love this one. Isn't this great advice? Don't touch amalgam, but go ahead and stuff it into every cavity you can find all day long. Aren't the tooth, tongue and cheeks of the patient in direct contact with the amalgam?

*Don't heat amalgam

"Mercury or amalgam should never be heated." [72]

Heated? Above what temperature? Freezing? Room temperature? Body temperature? 140 degrees? Hot coffee has been shown to heat fillings in the mouth up to near 140 degrees.

*Don't use mercury disinfecting solutions

"The use of mercury disinfecting solutions should be eliminated ..."
73

The ADA says not to use mercury disinfecting solutions because they are a source of mercury exposure. But it is okay with the ADA to use amalgam, a potentially much larger source of mercury exposure.

*Check dental clothing

"Clothing and shoes should be checked for mercury and amalgam before leaving the dental areas to avoid contamination of non-dental areas." 74

Now, please tell me how the average dentist is supposed to check for mercury on his or her clothes? Mercury has no taste. Mercury has no smell. Mercury vapor is invisible and often particles of amalgam arc too small to be visible.

Can you imagine your dentist checking his or her clothing and shoes before leaving the dental areas to avoid contaminating the non-dental areas?

Suppose the dentist does find mercury contamination? What then? Do they remove the contaminated shoes or clothing and get into new shoes or clothing before leaving the mercury work area? If the clothing or shoes are contaminated, special hazardous waste disposal guidelines should be followed.

The simplest solution to all these problems is to eliminate the use of mercury in the dental office. There is absolutely no need to have mercury in today's dental profession.

Dr. Hardy's "recommendations" in dental mercury hygiene

The ADA provides us with a flood of recommendations about mercury. I provide one: DON'T USE IT!

Imagine a dentist in practice, reading these ADA mercury recommendations. What are the reasons for these recommendations? Many were not taught in dental school of the potential hazards of mercury. Many were not taught what good office ventilation means or how often to change filters or even what type of air filters to use. If amalgam is safe in patients' mouths, why, for heavens' sake, must the left over part be stored under sulfuric acid in a tightly closed container? Why are there special hazardous waste disposal guidelines for one piece of amalgam, but the other piece (left in the patient's tooth) is safe? And why shouldn't a filling be touched that is being implanted daily into patients' bodies? Mercury is poisonous. That is the reason for all these recommendations.

Many dentists have not been taught how to properly dispose of mercury contaminated items. Even if they dispose of amalgam in a way which they think is proper, dentists can still be held liable for pollution caused by the amalgam. The next story illustrates my point.

58 Dentists pay for mercury clean up from amalgam, 1988

"Fifty-eight New England dentists have reached an out-of-court settlement with the Environmental Protection Agency (EPA) to pay partial damages in the cleanup of two sites where mercury contamination was found several years ago, the result of improperly processed amalgam." [75]

The dentists legally sold leftover amalgam to a salvage company that did not process the amalgam correctly, contaminating the soil.

According to the Superfund law, the dentists were held partly liable because they were the source of the amalgam. Two large areas were contaminated with mercury from the scrap amalgam. The EPA declared amalgam a hazardous substance and was able to find 58 dentists responsible for partial damages associated with the cleanup. Of course, if mercury was not used in dental fillings, this would have never happened. (For further details on this story, see story entitled Amalgams Declared Hazardous by EPA, page 161)

"60 Minutes" airs amalgam woes, 1990

It was Sunday night December 16, 1990, and "60 Minutes" was on the air. The lead piece that night, on dental mercury amalgam, was titled, "Is There a Poison in Your Mouth?" Several people were interviewed who had remarkably recovered from serious illnesses such as multiple sclerosis and arthritis after removing their mercury fillings. One woman said that the day after her amalgams were removed, she tossed her walking cane at her incredulous doctor and went out dancing that night.

Now, it may seem obvious to many that it is impossible for a poison to be eliminated from the body within 24 hours. But the problems with mercury fillings are not limited to the poison mercury. The fillings act like little batteries and radio antennas inside our heads. So, the relief this particular woman experienced could well have been the instant removal of the batteries and radio antennas that were her fillings. Once an electrical interference is removed from the body, it is gone. There is no lingering elimination time. (See BEM page 142.)

It was a fair and insightful news report on the amalgam controversy. The story made the public aware of the dangers in the continued use of dental amalgam. The great silence, the ADA's great taboo of telling the public about the controversy had been broken. And it was broken by one of the most respected and watched news magazine programs of this century.

The ADA went into a tizzy. No greater effort has ever been undertaken by the ADA to undermine, confuse and defuse the mercury controversy. The "60 Minutes" story reached millions of viewers in a single evening, catapulting the issue into sudden and high prominence. Intimidation, vague charges of ethics violations and attempts at brainwashing were the trademarks of the ADA's disinformation campaign.

"Special Report" distributed by the ADA, 1991

The ADA wrote a letter of protest to the "60 Minutes" staff and top network executives at CBS, the network that aired the show.

Then, it inserted a six-page booklet entitled "Special Report" in the January 1991 edition of the *Journal of the American Dental Association*. It had a cover letter from the ADA president, addressed to members. The subjects in the booklet were the ethics of removing amalgam, what the ADA felt "60 Minutes" should have covered, an overview of amalgam and mercury and sound bites from member dentists and from the Canadian Dental Association.

The ADA president said that the report had all the answers dentists needed for any patient question about the "60 Minutes" broadcast. The president's letter included permission to photocopy and hand out the information to patients. But, when I requested permission to use quotes from that handout in this book, I was denied. Of what are they afraid?

You see, most ADA members don't know much about mercury and its adverse health effects because it is not a subject taught in dental school, even though amalgam is by far the most widely used restorative in dentistry. Most information the typical dentist receives on the mercury issue has been filtered through the ADA.

Naturally the ADA wants to protect its interests. It's scary to me when a national organization starts telling its members what to say and, by inference, what to believe.

In the "Special Report," the ADA president said that state and local dental societies and dental schools were all given information put together by the ADA for their use in discussions with the public, the profession and the news media. Is it the ADA's job to also tell schools and dental societies what to say and, by inference, what to believe? Isn't there enough intelligence in those institutions to allow them to think for themselves?

The ADA president's letter also said that the ADA had put together a video news release and a radio release and beamed it to thousands of American radio and TV stations. The releases contained information on the safety of amalgam and were intended to quiet any suggestions that amalgam was a health risk. The ADA attempted to limit the damage by circulating their biased point of view on amalgam.

Ethics and big brother ADA

In the ethics section of the "Special Report," the ADA said that the dentist, using his or her best judgment, who removes amalgams from the non-allergic patient for the purpose of removing toxic substances from the body is acting improperly and unethically. The report also said that the dentist who removes amalgam from anybody who requests it, is not acting unethically. And the dentist who does not comply with the patient's request is not acting unethically, unless the amalgam removal was requested by a physician.

So now, let's review what the ADA is telling us is ethical vs. unethical in amalgam removal:

Chapter 3

Ethical to the ADA

It's OK to remove mercury amalgams if a patient wants it done, even though most patients have no medical background to make such a determination for their health, other than what they have heard and read.

It's OK to place a known poison, mercury, in patient's mouths, even though we are telling you not to touch the filling with your bare hands.

It's OK to refuse to remove amalgam, if the patient alone requests it.

Unethical to the ADA

It's not OK for the medically trained and tested professional, the dentist, to make an educated determination as to what is best for his/her patient's health. In other words, it is not ethical for a dentist, according to the ADA, to decide if a patient could benefit from mercury removal. The ADA says it is unethical for a knowledgeable and health-conscious dentist to decide to remove mercury, a poisonous substance, from patients' teeth.

Just for the record, it's not up to the ADA to tell me what is best for my patients. This is its current position. But I am a trained and qualified professional. I have come to an independent and different conclusion: The ADA does not have the power to dictate policies and procedures to member dentists, much less to non-members. But the ADA has a long arm. Most dentists who are members of license review boards are members of the ADA. So, the ADA has influence over legal actions against those opposed to its views. But this is, after all, a democracy, founded upon differences of opinion.

There follows even more astounding comments contained in the 1991 "Special Report."

Fairy tales from the ADA, or, What the ADA says "60 Minutes" should have told you

ADA fairy tale #1:
Amalgam is not a significant source of mercury exposure. Food, water and air are more significant sources than amalgam and everyone is exposed to these.

The truth is:
One of the most respected international authorities on mercury, Thomas W. Clarkson, Ph.D., M.D., of the University of Rochester says:

"The release of mercury from dental amalgams makes the predominant contribution to human exposure to inorganic mercury including mercury vapor in the general population." [76]

In simpler terms, dental mercury amalgams are the most significant source of mercury exposure for the general public.

And the World Health Organization in 1991 found that the major source of the body's stored mercury also came from dental amalgams. [77]

Even if the ADA was partly correct, which they aren't, it doesn't make medical sense to expose anyone to more mercury through their fillings, especially if they are already exposed to it in food, water and air.

ADA fairy tale #2:
Because of their exposure to mercury, dentists and dental staff would be more likely to show ill effects from it. But, according to the ADA's Special Report, dentists are in as good or better health than the average person.

Chapter 3

The truth is:
The ADA's own newspaper of August 13,1984, contradicts this very statement. Dr. Bernard P. Tillis writes in his letter titled "Doctor, Heal Thyself:"

"Cardiovascular disease, neuromuscular disturbances, gastrointestinal, respiratory and dermatologic complications are said to occur more frequently among dentists than in the average individual . . . Surveys, although not yet definitive, seem to indicate a suicide rate among dentists well above that of the general public . . . (these surveys) should become the stimuli for self-evaluation by each practitioner. The causes of stress can be determined! Is my staff inadequate? Am I undertaking projects beyond my present capacities? Are the operatories too confining? Are irritating gases or mercury present in the operatory?" [78]

The ADA should read its own newspaper once in a while.

ADA fairy tale #3:
Mercury exposure happens all the time. Many trace metals are required for good health and mercury is a trace metal. [79]

The truth is:
This assertion, found in the ADA Special Report is expressed by Dr. Stamm, dean of the School of Dentistry at the University of North Carolina at Chapel Hill. He completely and intentionally misleads the reader into assuming that mercury could be a part of a healthy diet. He might as well have said the same of lead. There is no use for mercury or lead in our diet.

Dr. Stamm never clearly says that trace amounts of mercury are required for good health, because he knows that is false. But words like "commonplace" and "routine" and "essential" are carefully chosen to convey safety and normality. There is nothing commonplace about being exposed to a serious poison. There is nothing routine about mercury exposure. There is nothing essential to health that includes a daily intake of mercury.

Composites: superior to amalgam

Composite resin fillings are the replacement material for amalgam. They are composed in large part of quartz or a silicon powder and a resin matrix in which the particles are suspended. The truth is that today many composites are superior to amalgam. A 1994 study by the prestigious Clinical Research Associates group of Provo, Utah, looked at 21 dental filling materials over three years. They ranked each according to wear, marginal adaptation (closeness of fit to the tooth), surface smoothness, wear of opposing teeth, breakage and color match.

Eleven of the 21 filling materials are composites used for fillings. They are called direct placement composite resins. The ADA and its members have been saying for years that direct placement composite resins are inferior to amalgam because they wear faster, have more recurrent decay and may increase the need for root canals. The Provo study demonstrated that all of these claims are untrue.

The results showed that recurrent decay and root canal therapy did not happen often enough on all materials combined to even be considered as significant. Amalgam was ranked 14th in overall strength, durability and effectiveness behind 11 composite filling materials and two porcelain/ceramic materials. Ten of the top 11 materials were composites. Almost two-thirds of the materials studied were found to be superior to amalgam. [80]

I have 14-year-old composite resins in my mouth and they are doing fine. They are in the highest stress-bearing teeth in my mouth, my molars. Similar results are seen on many patients. I still treat the very first patient I saw as a practicing dentist. She still has the composites I placed in her teeth nearly 14 years ago. The fillings are still doing well.

Do you want an inferior mercury amalgam, or a superior composite resin? The choice is yours, not the dentist's.

Now we know what the ADA says about mercury exposure from amalgam. What does our own government say about the standards for mercury exposure in the general population?

U.S. Government standards for mercury exposure

The recommended standard for occupational exposure to inorganic mercury applies to mercury exposure in the dental office. The National Institute for Occupational Safety and Health recommends the following procedures be adhered to for workers occupationally exposed to all organic and inorganic mercury compounds except methyl and ethyl mercury compounds:

*Comprehensive medical examinations before the employee starts and annually thereafter.

These exams are to emphasize the signs and symptoms of mercury exposure such as weight loss, insomnia, tremors, personality changes, or other symptoms of central nervous system exposure. These records are to be kept by the employer for five years after the employee's last exposure to inorganic mercury. [81]

It would be a safe bet that a survey of dental offices across the United States would find few, if any, offices that have done this medical testing.

*Warnings must be posted at entrances to areas where there is a potential exposure to mercury.

The warnings should read:[82]

```
WARNING!
MERCURY
HIGH CONCENTRATIONS
ARE HAZARDOUS TO HEALTH
MAINTAIN ADEQUATE VENTILATION
```

Warnings in mercury work areas are to read:[83]

```
WARNING!
MERCURY WORK AREA
UNAUTHORIZED PERSONS
NOT PERMITTED
```

I have never seen these signs in a dental facility of any kind. How would you feel if these signs were posted in the lobby of your dental office and in each treatment room? These are the federal government recommendations, yet the dental profession has not complied.

*Workers exposed to mercury shall be provided full body work clothing, such as coveralls, shoes or shoe covers and hats worn during work hours. Work clothing is to be vacuumed before removing. There is to be a separate locker for work clothes and street clothes. Workers are to shower before changing into street clothes.[84]

I can't remember a dentist or a dental assistant ever wearing coveralls, shoe covers and a hat. And I know of not one that showers and changes clothes before leaving work because he or she is exposed to mercury.

*Floors, work surfaces and equipment should be designed to have no cracks, crevices or any area that can retain mercury, such as carpeting.[85]

There must be thousands of dental offices in the U.S. that have carpeting in the treatment rooms. Most of them use mercury daily.

*Vacuums used in mercury work areas must have special mercury-absorbing filters. Compressed air cannot be used to blow mercury off equipment because it disperses mercury throughout the work area. With rare exception, all dental drills and air syringes work off compressed air. When drilling out an old amalgam, high levels of mercury vapor can be generated and spread throughout the operatory. The common practice of using the air syringe to blow off the counters and chairs may also spread mercury vapor.

*Mercury exposure levels should be regularly monitored.[86]

Does your dentist work with mercury? If so, does your dentist have a mercury-absorbing filter on the vacuum? And does your dentist monitor mercury levels in the office?

"Because mercury can cling to clothing and other items, the worker should be extremely careful about personal hygiene. A worker can easily carry mercury home on clothing, on the hands and under the fingernails. The mercury can then vaporize, or be eaten, adding to the worker exposure and possibly endangering his or her family as well ."[87]

". . . No food or tobacco should be kept or used in areas where mercury is present." [88]

No food is to be used in areas where mercury is present. But, it's okay to chew down with 14 tons of pressure on fillings that continuously release mercury?

14 Tons

When eating, average biting pressures of 170-200 pounds per square inch are reached. If 170 pounds per square inch of pressure is applied to the tip of a tooth that has an area of 6 thousandths of a square inch, the pressure concentrates for a total of 28,000 pounds.[89] Fourteen tons is a lot of pressure! Why don't teeth break more often? Because tooth enamel has an average compressive strength of 55,000 pounds per square inch.[90] Enamel can take the pressure. But that amount of pressure creates friction and heat. Friction and heat from chewing on amalgams increases the amount of mercury vapor released and scrapes tiny particles off the surface. So, the more one chews, the more mercury one breathes and swallows. Composite resin fillings have no mercury. No matter how hard you chew on the new composites, they will not release mercury.

An important, yet obscure danger in using amalgam lies in what many dentists paint the tooth with prior to the mercury fillings being inserted. That substance is called cavity varnish. It is composed of a natural gum or a synthetic resin dissolved in chloroform, ether or acetone.[91] This is painted directly on the tooth and the solvent evaporates into the patient's mouth.

Amalgams will become history

Back in the days when amalgam was created, most dentists had few, if any, qualifications to be a dentist. The few respectable dental practitioners and those with scientific backgrounds recognized mercury fillings as poisonous. However, the overwhelming numbers of those using mercury amalgam drowned out the voices of medical prudence and reason. The ADA, formed by those who used mercury amalgam, is so intrinsically linked to promoting and justifying amalgam, it can be argued that if there was never mercury amalgam, there would be no ADA.

We've seen how the ADA vehemently insists that a known poison, mercury, magically ceases to be itself in the mouth. And we've seen how governmental recommendations concerning mercury exposure are ignored in dental offices.

How long will this go on? I believe when the average dental consumer understands the risks associated with mercury in fillings, amalgams will become history.

Personal health risks are outlined and discussed in the next chapter. It may astound you.

4

master of

disguise

Mercury-A Universe Of Trouble

Master of disguise

Mercury, the mysterious silver liquid known as quicksilver, brings with its shiny countenance sickness and disease. Throughout centuries, man has sought to understand mercury's enigmatic charm. It has been only recently that we've realized the magnitude of its deception. Mercury has not brought a bevy of gifts as much as it has brought us a universe of trouble.

Mercury is the master element of disguise. It has no smell. It has no taste. It can enter the body as a vapor, a liquid or a solid. Once inside, it can change from one form to another, sneaking its way past the body's natural barriers and defenses.

Mercury has a detrimental effect on every organ system in the body. The smaller and younger you are, the more damage it can do. The unborn baby is especially vulnerable. Everything is affected: brain, kidneys, heart, lungs, stomach, intestines, mouth, blood vessels, liver, eyes, ears, skin, hormones, immune system, nervous system and even personality and behavior. The list of symptoms for mercury exposure is so long, it can be overwhelming. Over 200 different symptoms are found in medical literature. Most people reading the list would find it hard to believe that all these problems could be caused by one poison. Well, meet mercury, the master of disguise.

In this chapter, I briefly explain all the major body systems and the destructive effects mercury has on each. Mercury exposure symptoms mimic a host of common diseases for which there are currently no known cause. So, examples of these similarities and reasons why mercury exposure could be a factor in these and other disease progressions are brought to light.

The brain and central nervous system are major targets for mercury poisoning. Personality, behavioral and emotional effects are often the first signs of mercury toxicity. However, there are no useful tests to determine early stages of mercury toxicity for certain organ systems such as the nervous system.[92] This means there is no way to tell for sure what damage has already occurred in the brain until obvious symptoms appear such as tremors or memory and personality disturbances. It can sometimes take years or decades of low-level mercury exposure before these symptoms show up. Then, vague symptoms may begin to appear such as increasing anxiety, or fading short-term memory, or feeling more fatigued.

Why does it take so long to show up? Because low doses of mercury take time to accumulate in the body before reaching a critical tolerance level. When that level is reached, symptoms begin to appear. Tolerance levels vary from person to person. So, what might be safe for you, may not be safe for your son or daughter, or the neighbor down the street.

Mercury-induced health problems did not happen before man mined and used mercury. Which means that the naturally occurring levels of mercury did not pose a health problem, but the additional mercury exposure created by man's activities has.[93]

Before I present the specific health-related consequences of mercury exposure, I will summarize the three forms in which mercury presents itself. All three may be found in a person with amalgam fillings. Even though the major component of amalgam is metallic mercury, this kind of mercury can transform into the two other forms inside the body as a result of naturally occurring bacteria and chemical reactions. [94] All three forms of mercury are poisonous.

The three forms of mercury are; metallic, inorganic and organic. Most naturally occurring mercury is inorganic. Many man-made products contain metallic and organic mercury.

Metallic mercury (liquid)

Liquid mercury is metallic. It is an excellent electrical conductor and is as heavy and dense as lead. It is used in:
• Dental amalgam fillings
• Chlorine manufacturing
• Gold mining
• Electrical equipment (batteries, switches, thermostats, children and adult sport shoes that light up and trunk or hood lid light switches on cars)
• Instruments (thermometers, barometers)

Inorganic mercury

Mercury in combination with anything except carbon is called

inorganic. Inorganic mercury often comes as a powder. It can be white, red, yellow or black. It is used in:
- Electrical equipment (batteries, fluorescent bulbs, lamps)
- Cosmetics (certain red colors may contain mercuric oxides)
- Medicinal products (hemorrhoid ointments, merthiolate, mercurochrome, contact lens solutions; these last three products have been removed from the market)
- Tattoos (certain red colors)
- Vaccines, both for children and adults (as thimerosal, a preservative)

Organic mercury

Mercury in combination with carbon and anything else is called organic. Usually, this form of mercury is the most deadly. Often it is a powder or a liquid. It is found in:
- Contaminated fish and shellfish taken from polluted water
- Fungicides used in farming and seed preservation
- Paint preservatives

How does mercury get into the filling?

As we've learned, "amalgam" means a mixture of mercury and other metals. It is the dental term for the common "silver" filling. A liquid and powder are mixed vigorously to make the amalgam. The liquid is pure metallic mercury. The powder is a mixture of silver, tin, zinc or copper and other trace metals.

Mercury, you may recall, is by far the largest part of an amalgam, making up 50-70%. Some amalgams are pre-weighed and encapsulated ready for mixing right before placement in the cavity. Others are made by hand right next to the patient, using liquid mercury and metal powder dispensers.

Chapter 4

How does mercury escape from the filling?

As mercury amalgam fillings age in teeth, they break down. From the very second they are placed in the tooth until the last speck is removed, mercury, as vapor, is released. On a microscopic level, this loss of mercury creates tiny cracks and gaps in the structure of the filling, like craters on the moon or the deep cracks seen after an earthquake. These voids, defects and irregularities can eventually cause amalgams to break. Sometimes pieces chip off the edges; other times the entire filling falls out.

In addition to mercury vapor being released from the amalgam, small particles containing mercury are ground off the surface every time you chew. And corrosion, (the normal chemical and electrical reactions between food, liquids and amalgams happening 24 hours a day), releases even more mercury as vapor.

Some of the mercury that comes off from corrosion, chewing and the constant vaporization is combined with other molecules like chlorine. (Chlorine is found in tap water and in salt.) This creates inorganic mercury that can be transformed by naturally occurring bacteria into the more toxic organic mercury. This is why all three forms of mercury can be found in the person with mercury amalgam fillings.

If you have dental amalgam, then you are exposed to colorless, odorless and tasteless mercury 24 hours a day. Since there already is a certain level of naturally occurring mercury in our environment, your mercury exposure and its associated health risks increase with mercury amalgams.

Have you ever seen an ice cube tray come out of the freezer with tiny ice cubes where there should have been big ones? You can especially see this in frost-free freezers. What happens is that the water in the tray evaporates off the ice cubes and the cubes become smaller. This process -- evaporation off a solid -- is called sublimation. Mercury sublimes from fillings in much the same way water evaporates off ice cubes.

Mercury is the only metal that is liquid at room temperature. That is why it works so well in thermometers. For the most part, our bodies are also liquid, and inside the body, mercury atoms move around just as freely as almost any other liquid. That's why mercury can be detrimental to every organ system in the body.

Mercury fillings don't noticeably change shape because amalgam has a crystalline structure that keeps its shape even while losing weight. Mercury is extremely dense, so quite a lot can evaporate (sublime) off before any change can be seen, even microscopically. But if you've ever had a mercury filling crack or break, you know its structure is weakening.

Mercury is so dense that a droplet spilled in a room can saturate the air with mercury vapor in minutes. And the rest of the droplet still on the floor would take years to completely evaporate.

How much mercury comes off the filling?

The question of how much mercury comes off the filling is not as important as knowing that mercury continually comes off each and every amalgam. Even the smallest amounts can present a danger especially over years of exposure. However, it is important to seek answers.

The amount of mercury released from a filling depends on the newness of the amalgam, what other metals are present in the mouth, what oral habits are there (such as smoking, chewing, teeth clenching and grinding) and the types and temperatures of foods ingested.

The hotter water gets, the faster it evaporates as steam off the surface. The same is true for the mercury in your fillings. The warmer amalgams get, from the friction of chewing or the temperature of hot foods or smoking, the more mercury "boils" off the surface. You never know it, because mercury vapor, unlike steam, is invisible, odorless and tasteless. Studies show a large amount of mercury vapor is released from amalgams regardless of their age after only a few minutes of gum chewing.[95] Measurements of mercury vapor were eight times the maximum allowable average mercury concentration set for a 40-hour week by the National Institute for Occupational Safety and Health in 1973. One study demonstrated an increase in mercury vapor in people's mouths of 15,600% after chewing gum.[96] Who would think a stick of gum could be such a villain? Who would think a bowl of hot homemade soup or seven-grain bread could be unhealthy because of its heating up of the common "silver" fillings?

Maybe you have increased fiber in your diet because you have heard of its benefits in avoiding colon problems. Well, if you chew that increased fiber on amalgams, more mercury can be driven off due to the increased heat of friction. So, improving your diet may not always improve your health!

And if that isn't enough, when different types of metals are present in the mouth, more corrosion occurs, releasing even more mercury. Connecting gold to amalgams or amalgams to each other by braces or a partial denture can also increase the release of mercury.

How does mercury get into the body?

A quick review: Metallic mercury is liquid metal; inorganic mercury is often a powder containing mercury combined with anything except carbon; organic mercury (also often a powder) is mercury combined with carbon and anything else.

Metallic mercury vapor easily enters the body through the lungs. From there, it is rapidly transported by the bloodstream to other parts of the body. If swallowed, metallic mercury does not enter the bloodstream easily and can pass through the digestive system.

The major target organs for mercury vapor are the central nervous system and the kidneys. So, metallic mercury preferentially, but not exclusively, lodges in the brain and kidney.

Inorganic mercury is also absorbed through the lungs but not quite as quickly as the metallic form. However, inorganic mercury can pass directly through the skin and, if swallowed, enters the bloodstream more easily than metallic mercury. The favorite targets of inorganic mercury are the kidneys.

Organic mercury enters the body easily through the lungs. Once in your bloodstream, it is rapidly transported to other parts of your body. And, as with metallic mercury, its favorite resting places are the brain and kidneys. It can also enter directly through the skin, but not as quickly as inorganic mercury.[97]

What exactly does mercury do in the body?

Mercury causes trouble in the body, a universe of trouble. More than 200 signs and symptoms resulting from mercury exposure are cited in scientific literature. In this chapter, I will explore the most common of these. Let's look at the research.

Areas of mercury's harm: Birth Defects/ Reproductive Disorders

I was taught in dental school not to place mercury amalgams in pregnant women because of the possibility of toxic mercury effects on the fetus. How many women who don't know they are pregnant have mercury placed in their teeth each year? What effects can this have on the developing fetus?

Birth defects and reproductive disorders encompass what are probably some of the most sensitive medical issues. After all, children are our future, and their safety, as much as is possible, is truly our responsibility. Certainly, any hazard should be eliminated from our children's lives before and after they are born.

Developing fetuses are particularly susceptible to metallic mercury accumulation in the brain and kidneys because it readily crosses the placental barrier. The mercury vapor constantly released from

93

amalgams in the mother's teeth is from metallic mercury, the material used to make amalgams.

The hormone responsible for uterine contraction during labor and milk "letdown" for nursing is affected by exposure to low concentrations of mercury.[98] One certainly doesn't want to interfere with normal growth and development. And one positively, absolutely doesn't want to interfere with a woman in labor.

Chromosomes

Before a baby takes shape in the uterus, it is just half of mom's chromosomes and half of dad's chromosomes coming together to make the fertilized egg. This microscopic union produces a complex and wonderfully unique baby.

Just how significant are the chromosomes? Chromosomes are made up of DNA, a complex protein that within its double-helix shape contains all the genetic information for almost all forms of life. Genetic information encodes all the characteristics that make us individuals, such as hair, eye and skin color as well as all the other traits that we inherit. Chromosomes carry all the genetic messages from our parents. Alterations in chromosomes can produce devastating or fatal birth defects. Anything that can alter the structure of DNA can dramatically alter or even prevent life.

Mercury in all its forms can lodge in the fetus. Mercury vapor -- the kind that comes off amalgam fillings -- and organic mercury have been clearly shown to cause chromosome damage and induce numerous types of birth defects.[99] Mercury causes these defects by altering the structure of DNA. Studies have found that mercury compounds decrease the molecular weight of DNA and change the shape of the DNA helix.[100,101] Mercury is also known to inhibit the enzyme responsible for making the building blocks of DNA.[102]

Birth defects from organic mercury exposure include cleft palate, limb defects, brain and facial malformations, cerebral palsy, mental retardation and general growth retardation.[103]

Poisoned and didn't even know it

Cerebral palsy is a nonprogressive paralysis due to inhibited brain development from chemical exposure or trauma during birth. It can be a devastating result in pregnant women exposed to mercury. Too often, the women have no idea they are at risk at all. The difference in sensitivity to mercury toxicity for an adult versus a fetus is both dramatic and terrifying.

A tragic example of this occurred in Minamata Bay, Japan. For 36 years, beginning in 1932, the Chisso factory dumped an estimated total of 200-600 tons of mercury-laden waste into the bay. People living along the coastal area regularly ate fish from the polluted water. Babies were born with cerebral palsy, convulsions, slow reflexes, retarded body growth, speech disorders, mental retardation, limb deformities, hyperactivity, crossed eyes and spastic muscle twitching. Small heads were seen in 60% of the babies and the death rate was 7%. Most of the pregnant women exposed to the organic mercury showed no signs of poisoning. [104,105]

It was not until 1956, 24 years after the dumping began, that organic mercury poisoning was suggested as the cause of the tragedy. It took many more years to stop mercury waste dumping into the bay.[106] How many more years will it take for the dental profession to realize that mercury should not be used in human beings?

Biotransformation

Biotransformation refers to the conversion of one compound into another, commonly by bacteria. By now you know that mercury vapor rises off amalgam 24 hours a day. What you might not know is that this mercury vapor can be biotransformed into methylmercury.

Methylmercury is one of the most poisonous compounds known

to man. Its effects on the nervous system are profound and often permanent.[107] Since only metallic mercury is used in the making of an amalgam, it was thought that methylmercury exposure from amalgam was impossible.

However, in 1975, two studies showed that a variety of human intestinal bacteria and yeasts could create methylmercury from inorganic mercury.[108,109] And, even worse, in April 1983, research proved that mercury from amalgam was methylated to the potent methylmercury by common human mouth bacteria. [110]

Methylmercury is extremely toxic to adults and even more so in developing fetuses. Even though only a small amount of the mercury released from fillings may be methylated, how much is settling in the brain, the kidneys or the pregnant woman's child? No amount of methylmercury affects any child's development in a positive way.

Mercury has no place in human development. It has no beneficial effects on the human body, especially on a baby.

CARDIOVASCULAR (heart and blood vessels)

Studies have revealed important links between cardiovascular problems and mercury exposure. For instance, exposure to mercury vapor has been shown to increase blood pressure in humans. An increase in blood pressure can greatly increase the risk of heart attack or stroke, and heart attacks and strokes account for more than half the deaths each year in the United States. [111,112]

No amalgams, lower blood pressure

In an important study, a significant increase in blood pressure was found in volunteers with dental amalgam compared to a group that had no amalgam fillings. The group with mercury amalgams had blood pressure levels closer to the average reported for the general population. The group without amalgams had a lower blood pressure than the average for the general population. Amalgams have been estimated to be used in 75% to 80% of all tooth restorations. The study's author noted that the population from which the "normal" blood pressure was derived most likely had amalgam fillings. [113]

Possibly it wasn't the lack of amalgams, but something else, that caused the lower blood pressure. For instance, maybe the people who choose to be mercury-free are healthier than the general population and, therefore, already have lower blood pressure. On the other hand, maybe it was the lack of mercury fillings that lowered the blood pressure. Think of it . . . the "normal" U.S. blood pressure would be skewed by having so many people, 100 million, with mercury amalgams. What would the normal blood pressure be if no one had mercury amalgams? Would the average person have lower blood pressure and, therefore, a lower risk of heart trouble? This is an important, yet unanswered question.

Palpitations from fillings?

Exposure to mercury vapor has caused heart palpitations in humans. [114] Mercury vapor is the main type of human exposure from mercury fillings. The more amalgam fillings one has, the more the mercury exposure. Add different metals found in crowns, bridges or partials and one has even more mercury released from the amalgams. Maybe there is so little coming off the fillings that no symptoms show for a year, or even another year or the year after. How many years of accumulation does it take before it does affect the individual? How much mercury vapor can be breathed before getting high blood pressure or palpitations? No one can say. People react differently to mercury. Some have more resistance than others. But why risk it at all?

ENDOCRINOLOGICAL (hormones)

Hormones rule general body development and growth, food

metabolism, salt and water balance, sexual development and repro-
duction. If hormones are out of balance, especially in children, they
can do lifelong harm. Hormone imbalances can make a giant or a
dwarf. They can create hyperactivity or sluggishness and strong or
brittle bones. Hormonal disorders can cause diabetes insipidus, diabetes mellitus, hypoglycemia, hyperthyroidism, hypothyroidism, goiter, Addison's disease, Cushing's syndrome, osteoporosis and other
serious diseases.

Mercury exposure has been found to alter hormone levels by
interfering with the hormone-making glands, the endocrine glands.
Let's look briefly at some of these glands.

The body's mail carriers

Endocrine glands produce hormones. I think of hormones as the
body's mail carriers. The "master gland," or the main post office, is in
the brain. It is called the pituitary. Hormones are the body's chemical
mail, traveling from the master gland to other endocrine glands, finally arriving at their proper addresses with messages. These messages, if
correct, smoothly control major body functions. Incorrect, overly
weak, overly strong messages or no message at all, can be disruptive or
disastrous to the body.

The messenger, ironically, disrupts the mail

Mercury, the mythological being, was known as the messenger in
the Roman era. Mercury, the metal, ironically disrupts the body's mail
at many levels, interfering with the body's messages. It interferes with
the main post office, as well as the branch offices around the body.

Research shows that mercury is hard on hormones

In an exhaustive compilation of research on mercury toxicity done in the USSR, dysfunction of three major endocrine glands was noted. The thyroid, pituitary and adrenal glands were found to be adversely affected after exposure to very low concentrations of mercury.[115]

Both human and animal research show inorganic and organic mercury may alter hormone levels.[116] Amalgam gives off mostly metallic mercury vapor, but remember that some vapor can disguise itself by becoming inorganic mercury or organic mercury.

Thyroid

A 13-year-old boy exposed to mercury vapors for two weeks developed hyperthyroidism and his thyroid became enlarged. [117] Hyperthyroidism can result in goiter, rapid pulse, clammy skin, nervousness, palpitations, fatigue, increased appetite, weight loss, insomnia, weakness and frequent bowel movement. Its cause is listed as unknown.[118]

What if this teenager's mercury exposure went undiscovered? It certainly could have weakened his emotional stability, not to mention his physical status. A 13-year-old has enough personality changes to deal with. Mercury exposure only adds to the stress. How much does mercury exposure from amalgam contribute to the high rate of teen depression or suicide?

Pituitary, the master gland

The pituitary gland makes several hormones necessary for normal growth and development, and is therefore vitally important to children. It also secretes hormones responsible for water conservation by the kidneys.[119] Interference with water conservation may cause either edema (fluid retention and as a result, swelling) or dehydration, both of which could be life threatening. Mercury can create dysfunction of the pituitary gland, which in turn may interfere with these vital functions.[120]

Adrenal

The adrenal glands produce adrenalin for times of extreme stress when the "fight or flight" response is needed. Very low concentrations of mercury can cause adrenal dysfunction. When I call on the rush of adrenalin, I don't want to get a busy signal. So I am glad to be mercury-free.

Diabetes Mellitus

Diabetes Mellitus is characterized by high blood sugar levels resulting from either low insulin production or inactive (non-working) insulin. This type of diabetes is said to have no known cause. The longer one has the disease, the more it may result in increased risk of infection, heart attacks, gangrenous loss of limbs, blindness, numbness or paralysis in the feet and legs and kidney failure. In Diabetes Mellitus, there may be plenty of insulin in the blood, but it is not in what is called an active form.

Mercury inactivates the very enzyme that allows insulin to do its job.[121] After exposure to mercury, one may be left with plenty of insulin in the bloodstream, but much of it may be inactive. Long-term exposure to low levels of mercury may be a cause of Diabetes Mellitus.

Mercury may also interfere with insulin function by changing insulin's chemical shape. Active insulin has three sulfur bridges in its structure and sulfur is mercury's favorite element. Mercury may wedge itself into the sulfur bridges disrupting them and turning the active insulin inactive. The result again would be plenty of insulin circulating in the blood, but it would be inactive, just as seen in Diabetes Mellitus.

The beta cells of the pancreas produce insulin. Their destruction or impairment from organic mercury exposure may result in diabetes.

100

Remember, commonly found mouth and intestinal bacteria can turn mercury vapor from dental amalgam into organic mercury.

Autopsies of victims of Minamata disease, caused by ingestion of organic mercury, revealed some disintegration of the alpha and beta cells in the pancreas.[122]

In a country where diabetes is fairly common, we can ill afford to toss the monkey wrench of mercury exposure from dental fillings into the hormonal machinery. What are the effects of amalgam fillings on those with diabetes? How much does the constant low-level mercury exposure from these fillings contribute to the creation of diabetes?

FERTILITY/ PREGNANCY/LABOR COMPLICATIONS/ SPONTANEOUS ABORTIONS

In animal studies, mercury exposure has been shown to diminish sexual activity, lower sperm production and lower fertility.[123,124,125,126] Research has demonstrated time and time again that if it can happen in animals, it can happen in humans.

Mercury vapor is the main type of exposure from amalgam. In a 1980 study, women exposed to mercury vapor had increased rates of pregnancy and labor complications compared to unexposed women. And the effects were related to the length of exposure and concentration of mercury vapors.[127]

A study in Denmark showed increased rates of spontaneous abortion in a group of dental assistants working with mercury.[128]

Another study, done on Polish dental workers, also discovered an increased rate of spontaneous abortion from occupational mercury exposure.[129] Most dental assistants in the U.S. are women. What is the hazard level for each and every one of these women who work with mercury? Are dental offices required to be monitored for good mercury hygiene? No, they are not.

One woman exposed to mercury vapor reported that her first pregnancy ended in spontaneous abortion and her second baby died shortly after birth. When her exposure to mercury vapor ended and the obvious signs of mercury poisoning subsided, she produced a healthy child.[130]

Future fathers, beware!

Metallic mercury is the type of mercury used to make amalgam: A 1991 study showed that the rate of spontaneous abortions increased significantly in a group of mothers when the fathers were exposed to metallic mercury before the pregnancy. [131]

The fathers! This is truly disturbing. It means that men exposed to metallic mercury can increase the rate of women's spontaneous abortions. And the mothers may not be exposed to mercury at all except through contact with the fathers. A man's workplace can adversely affect the future of the family, the not-yet-conceived. The connection between mercury exposure in the mother and an increase in spontaneous abortions seems fairly obvious, but to suspect that fathers were such carriers of bad news is a surprise. Mercury is truly the master of disguise.

GASTROINTESTINAL (stomach and intestines)

Mercury exposure can cause anorexia, colitis, abdominal cramps, diarrhea, nausea and vomiting. When an infant died of fluid in his lungs after breathing mercury vapor, the autopsy indicated the lining of his stomach and duodenum (the first part of the small intestine connecting to the stomach) was dead.[132] Breathing mercury vapor affects not just the stomach and intestines but also the emotional connections we have with food and eating.

Anorexia nervosa occurs most frequently in teenage girls. However, it is not limited to teenagers. It is characterized by an extreme fear of becoming overweight, even when the person is grossly underweight. The popular musician Karen Carpenter died from this all-too-common affliction.

A 1976 report detailed how within two weeks teenage girls exposed to mercury vapor exhibited anorexia, intermittent abdominal cramps, diarrhea and painful bleeding gums.[133] It is disturbing to read that mercury vapor exposure can cause any form of anorexia. There is a huge psychological component to anorexia nervosa, which is potentially fatal and one of the most difficult teenage disorders to treat. Unfortunately, mercury vapor exposure also is known to have psychological components ranging from shyness and timidity to depression and anxiety.

In 1992, the Centers for Disease Control reported that most fillings in children are placed between the ages of 9 and 15.[134] It may be more than a coincidence that this age range closely parallels that of anorexia nervosa sufferers. Awkward teenage self-consciousness may be compounded by the mercury fillings. What if there is enough mercury released by the amalgam fillings inside a child's body to set the stage for anorexia? What if the last filling depresses the child just enough to start the cycle of self destruction? In how many cases has mercury from fillings been the snowflake that has caused the avalanche? The implications are grim.

Colitis, also known as irritable bowel syndrome (IBS), is an inflammation of the intestines. Symptoms may include mild to severe abdominal pain, constipation or diarrhea, fever, bleeding from the rectum and bloating following a meal. IBS represents about 50% of all gastrointestinal complaints or referrals. Anatomically, no cause for IBS has been found. Antibiotic therapy and amoebic infection (caused by a one-celled animal form of life found in some soil and water) are two known causes.[135,136] Ironically, abdominal pain and colitis are both symptoms listed under mercury poisoning in the most widely used manual of medical diagnosis and therapy, the Merck Manual.[137] Persons who have colitis should not have any exposure to mercury, no matter how small. Amalgams should not be used in colitis patients.

People with IBS can experience great pain. Stress (depression, anxiety, mood swings, insomnia, exposure to drugs or chemicals, fatigue and food allergies) can initiate or worsen an attack. Mercury exposure can cause depression, anxiety, mood swings, insomnia and fatigue. So, mercury exposure can certainly worsen IBS.

Initial symptoms of IBS (bloating, gas, nausea, headache, fatigue, depression, anxiety and difficulty in concentration) are commonly triggered by eating.[138] Every one of these symptoms is also a symptom of mercury exposure. Let's chew on that for a moment. Eating is the common trigger of IBS symptoms. Eating on mercury fillings puts pressure and friction on them, heating them up. This can greatly increase the mercury vapor released. Recall that one study demonstrated an increase in mercury vapor after chewing of 15,600% over resting levels.[139] Eating may be the trigger of IBS because amalgams heat up and release more mercury!

I have had patients with colitis request that their mercury fillings be replaced. Because there is a temporary increase in mercury vapor exposure during removal, each one had their symptoms flare up immediately after each removal session. However, subsequent visits produced less symptoms and in every case, the patients have had dramatically fewer colitis flare-ups since their amalgams were replaced by composite resins.

Sulfasalazine is a sulfur-containing drug long used for colitis. It is being used more frequently for treating rheumatoid arthritis.[140] (see Arthritis section, page 110) Sulfur, you may remember, is mercury's favorite element -- it attracts mercury strongly. I believe the reason why this drug works in colitis and arthritis is that it removes mercury from the body's tissues. (see Dr. Hardy's Arthritis Theory, page 111).

Remember, most amalgams in children are placed between age 9 and 15. Low-level mercury exposure, the kind you receive from amalgams, is cumulative over time. Most IBS/colitis cases occur between age 15 and 30.[141]

There are too many coincidences to be ignored. How many colitis victims have mercury amalgams? When did their symptoms begin? Do they notice flare-ups when they get a new amalgam? How many cases exist of colitis remission after amalgam removal?

Crohn's disease is very similar to IBS, with similar symptoms, triggers and treatment. Its cause is unknown. Colitis and Crohn's disease are so similar that, in some cases, knowing which is which may be difficult or impossible.

Most cases of Crohn's disease occur between the ages of 14 and 24,[142] allowing plenty of time for mercury vapor exposure from childhood amalgam fillings. It seems clear that people suffering from Crohn's disease or IBS would be better off without mercury entering their bodies via amalgam fillings.

HEMATOLOGICAL (blood)

Blood is composed of fluid (called plasma), red blood cells, white blood cells, platelets, fat globules, carbohydrates, proteins, hormones and gases.[143]

Proteins in the blood are crucial to blood pressure and the balance of fluids between the blood and the body. Mercury can interfere with nearly every protein function.

Mercury loves sulfur, which is in nearly every protein and is important in almost all protein functions. Mercury can attach to the sulfur found in proteins. In this way, nearly every protein in the body may be disrupted.[144]

The red blood cells carry oxygen to the body and bring carbon dioxide, the body's waste gas, back to the lungs for exhaling. Mercury can attach itself to every sulfur group found on the surface of red cells. This lowers the red cell's ability to carry oxygen and carbon dioxide.[145] This disturbance in the red cells may result in fatigue, a common symptom of mercury exposure.

The white blood cells protect the body against invaders such as bacteria, viruses, parasites and toxins. High frequencies of chromoso-mal abnormalities have been observed in white blood cells from humans exposed to mercury. [146,147,148,149] Chromosome aberrations can destroy the vital protective ability of white blood cells.

The neutrophils normally make up about two thirds of all white blood cells. They are the most active cells in the body's defense and are responsible for much of the body's protection against infection.[150] When neutrophils get too numerous, they can become involved in tissue destruction. We see this in various disorders called autoim-mune diseases such as rheumatoid arthritis, Diabetes Mellitus, colitis and AIDS.[151] Following exposure to mercury vapor, a moderate to high white blood cell count with a large increase in the neutrophils has been reported.[152,153]

Hemoglobin is the iron-containing molecule in the red blood cells. It is responsible for carrying oxygen from the lungs to the rest of the body and carbon dioxide back to the lungs.

A 1990 study concluded that participants with dental amalgam showed significantly decreased hemoglobin and numbers of red blood cells compared to those that had no dental amalgams.[154] Such decreases may result in anemia and fatigue.

Platelets are needed to form the blood clots that stop bleeding after an injury. An important enzyme required in the normal blood clotting process, called Factor XIIIa, is inhibited by mercury.[155]

Platelet membranes ruptured when they were exposed to the mercury-containing preservative thimerosal.[156] Thimerosal (known as Mercurochrome and Merthiolate) was removed by the FDA from the market due to ineffectiveness, but it is still put into many vaccines given to infants and adults. (See "Children's Vaccines Contain Mercury!" page 146)

The phrase "our life blood" exemplifies the importance of blood and its components. Our quality of life depends on the quality of our blood. This is the liquid of life. Why pollute this most important stream with mercury?

HEPATIC (liver)

The liver filters, cleans, detoxifies, manufactures and stores. It makes proteins found in the blood, stores glucose and stores vitamins B12, A, D, E and K. It regulates the amount of blood the body has and is one of the main sources of body heat. The liver makes fibrinogen, an important component of the blood clotting system and is also involved in fat metabolism.[157]

Serious liver problems in animals have been noted with high mercury vapor exposure, decreasing in severity as the dose decreases.[158] In humans, degenerative liver changes were noted in a young child exposed to mercury vapor.[159]

The liver is too important to one's well being to insult by knowingly making it work harder. We know mercury constantly escapes from each amalgam. We also know mercury creates problems with the blood. These problems must be cleaned up by the liver.

IMMUNOLOGICAL (body defenses)

The presence of dental amalgam may increase the risk of infectious disease, cancer and autoimmune diseases.

What is the immune system?

The immune system's job is to defend our body from bacteria, viruses and parasites as well as from chemical and physical injury. The part of our immune system called our natural immunity is thought to be relatively permanent and present at birth. However, babies' immune systems are not fully developed at birth, leaving the infants more susceptible to sickness and disease. Natural immunity may be determined by the individual's genes, diet and differences in metabolism. Other types of immunity are developed by the body through mother's milk, vaccines and exposure to organisms in daily living.

Our body's defense is carried out by white blood cells, proteins, blood vessels and chemicals. This defensive system is found everywhere in the body, from the skin to the intestines, from the eyes to the toes. When it is suppressed, it simply can't do its job as well. So when you hear the diagnosis of "immune-suppressed," it can be very serious. An immune-suppressed individual is more susceptible to infection, injury and disease.[160]

T cells

Because of the AIDS epidemic, referred to now as HIV infection, most people have heard of T cells. They are white blood cells that have been activated or modified by the thymus, hence the name, T cells. T cells are an important part of the immune system that deals with autoimmune disorders (more about these soon), cancer and viral, bacterial, yeast, fungal and other infections.[161] The ideal percentage of T cells found in the white blood cell population is between 70 and 80%.[162]

There was a report published in the *Journal of Prosthetic Dentistry* in May 1984, that described two patients whose T cell counts rose dramatically after amalgam fillings were removed.[163]

One patient, a 35-year-old woman, had a significant medical history including advanced multiple sclerosis (MS). She began the study with nine mercury amalgam fillings. Before the fillings were removed, her T cell percentage was 60%. After removal, the T cells rose to 71%.

The other patient was a 21-year-old woman in apparently good health. She began the study with six amalgam fillings. Before the amalgams were removed, her T cell percentage was 47%. After removal, the T cells rose to 73%, a 55.3% increase. This is dramatic, but what happened next was even more amazing. Four amalgams were put back into this 21-year-old. Her T cells decreased to 55%, a drop of 24.7%. When these amalgams were removed, her T cells again rose to 72%.[164]

These results strongly suggest that the presence of dental amalgam may lower the T cell count, which, in turn, increases the risk of infection, cancer and autoimmune diseases. Why take the chance?

B cells

Another type of white blood cell, the B cell, produces immunity for the body. B cells arise from the bone marrow, hence the name. Mercury exposure can suppress the B cells, further reducing our ability to combat disease and infection.[165]

Immunoglobulins are a family of related, but not identical, proteins which are important in our immune system. The most common one found in plasma is called IgG. IgG is the major defense against toxins, viruses and bacteria. And IgG gives immunity to the fetus before birth. Another immunoglobulin, called IgA, is the main defense in mucosa. Mucosa is what lines the mouth, nose sinuses, eyelids, lungs, vagina and intestines. IgA is thought to protect us from bacteria and viruses invading these mucosal surfaces.[166]

Two 1990 studies demonstrated that IgG levels decreased significantly in workers exposed to mercury vapor compared to those who were not exposed. One of the two studies also showed a significant decrease in IgA levels as well.[167,168]

How much mercury vapor from fillings affects our T cells, B cells and immunoglobulins is unclear. But mercury vapor can only have a negative effect on the body protectors.

Antibiotic-resistant infections

Mercury released from dental amalgam may contribute to the increase of antibiotic-resistant bacteria in humans.

Antibiotics are not working as well as they used to. As you may well imagine, this is considered a major problem in medicine today. The reason is the spread of antibiotic-resistant, disease-causing bacteria in humans. An increasing number of health professionals feel that antibiotics are over prescribed.

For the past 20 years, medical researchers have been baffled over why so much resistance is found. Previous evidence linked a person's recent use of antibiotics with his/her increased antibiotic resistance. But that did not explain the resistance found in those people who had no recent antibiotic use. Researchers discovered that people with a lot of mercury-resistant bacteria in their intestines were significantly more likely to also have bacteria resistant to two or more antibiotics.[169]

According to *Dentistry Today,* May 1993, "Mercury leaching from amalgam fillings appears to encourage the growth of bacteria that are resistant to antibiotics, as well as mercury." [170] When someone has an illness like strep throat or bronchitis and finds that the prescribed antibiotic is not working, he/she may be dealing with antibiotic-resistant bacteria and may be sicker for a longer time. Maybe he/she also has some amalgam fillings. How much are those fillings contributing to the protracted illness? Are extra work days being missed because of the fillings?

A 1991 study of 383 people for nearly three years showed a strong link between the presence of amalgam and extra work days missed. The number of days missed from work was compared the year before amalgam removal and one and two years after. The results indicate a 30% drop in sick days two years after amalgam removal.[171] What would be the savings in the U.S. of a 30% drop in sick leave among workers?

Rheumatoid Arthritis (RA)

Rheumatoid arthritis (RA) is a chronic, systemic, inflammatory disease of the joints. Pain, swelling and crippling distortion of the joints are common. Anyone who has RA or has known someone who has it, knows the debilitating pain. The cause of RA is unknown.[172,173]

Dr. Hardy's Arthritis (RA)/MS Theory

I have a theory that explains how mercury can create joint pain, arthritis-type symptoms and demyelination (loss of insulation) of nerve fibers such as are seen in Multiple Sclerosis. Nearly every medical student carries around a copy of the Merck Manual, a little green book that contains summaries of all known diseases, causes and treatments. The advertisement on the side of the packaging it comes in says "The world's most widely used comprehensive medical reference."

When I looked up RA and MS in the Merck Manual, I found the causes of each listed as unknown. RA is considered an autoimmune disease of connective tissue. The suspected cause of MS is an autoimmune disease of the insulation of the brain and spinal cord. This means that the body suddenly recognizes the connective tissue or insulation as abnormal and attacks it with what is called the inflammatory process. I believe this label of an autoimmune disease is incorrect (See Dr. Hardy's Theory on Autoimmune Diseases, page 121)

Joints and the outer coats of nerves' insulation are largely made up of connective tissue called collagen. Two collagen molecules are hooked together by two sulfur atoms, one from each molecule. The sulfur from one collagen holds the hand of the sulfur from another collagen forming a cross-link.

You've heard about sulfur before -- it is mercury's favorite atom. Well, mercury has a great affinity for two sulfur atoms at a time because it often has an electrical need for two. This means it can easily get in between the two sulfur atoms, holding each of their hands.

Once the normal connective tissue has one or more atoms of mercury between the sulfur atoms, that tissue is seen by the immune system as foreign tissue. This sets off a chain reaction called the inflam-

111

matory reaction against the "foreign" collagen with the mercury atoms. It then appears as if the body is attacking itself, hence the label autoimmune disease.

All of us who have gotten a splinter in our finger know of the swelling and redness that occur. This is the body's inflammatory reaction to the splinter being inside the finger. The mercury acts like a splinter in the collagen causing the reaction seen in RA joints and insulation-destroying nerve disorders such as Multiple Sclerosis.

RA treatment

There is further support for my RA/MS theory found in some treatments for RA. A common treatment is a drug called penicillamine. The <u>Merck Manual</u> says that when it is given orally, it may produce a beneficial effect on RA. Penicillamine is also commonly used in patients that have mercury poisoning. I find that more than a coincidence. So many of my patients find relief from arthritis when they become mercury-free and the same symptoms that apply to arthritis are found in mercury poisoning.

Another treatment for RA is gold compounds containing a small amount of sulfur. Mercury has such a strong attraction for gold that it has been used to mine gold for centuries. In the gold mining process, mercury is used to draw out the specks of gold from the mud slurry.

The reason gold relieves arthritis is unknown. I believe gold works by plucking out mercury atoms from between the sulfur atoms in the connective tissue. In this way, the connective tissue that was formerly seen as foreign reverts to normal, causing the inflammatory process to stop.

Most dramatic success with arthritis

In the 12 years I have been a mercury-free, health-centered dentist, the most dramatic success stories have been those patients with RA and chronic headaches. Nearly all with RA who replaced their amalgams have had improvement in their symptoms. Some improved only a bit, but most have recovered either dramatically, or completely. The amount of recovery seemed to depend on the length of time the disease had been present and, as I believe do most disease processes, on eating habits, exercise and general outlook on life.

A remarkable recovery

You may find interesting the following letter from one of my patients who came to me with RA.

To whom it may concern:

Approximately three years ago I began experiencing constant pain in my feet, then it progressed to my arms, elbows and hands. The pain was an aching type of pain deep in my muscles and joints, like a toothache. When I got out of bed in the morning I could hardly walk because my body was so stiff.

After seeing three different doctors, I was diagnosed as having rheumatoid arthritis because I had the same symptoms. My doctor prescribed medicine that helped me feel better right away and also a medication that took a long time to be effective (six months or longer). This medication was 'gold capsules.'

In the meantime, I saw the '60 Minutes' segment on television concerning mercury fillings. I had never heard or seen any information on 'Mercury Toxicity' from tooth fillings before. (I was 42 years old at the time!) Because I had a lot of mercury fillings, I decided that it would be worth my time, effort and money (to me) to have these fillings replaced with a safer composite. I had everything to gain and nothing to lose. I wanted my health back!

After having my mercury fillings replaced, I felt better and after detoxifying my body of its mercury burden, I felt even better. My blood work reflected that the amount of infection in my body had dropped back down within the normal range.

The gold capsules were decreased to half the dosage, then discontinued entirely. As of this date, I continue to experience improved health compared to three years ago. I still experience some mild symptoms which I feel is due to irreversible damage that has been done to my body.

Pat Taylor
Florida

A letter from her rheumatologist described her condition as he saw it. Although he remains unconvinced that her fillings actually caused her arthritis, he wrote that since Pat had been replacing her mercury amalgams, she had improved remarkably. He ended the letter by saying that her arthritis was in remission. The letter was unusual for two reasons. One, he had the courage to write the letter and two, he had the willingness to leave the door open on the possibility of mercury causing toxic problems in some individuals. He seems to be an astute physician who knows that we can learn much from listening to and clearly observing our patients.

As far as I understand, there is no known cure for rheumatoid arthritis and remission is rare. My guess is that mercury played a large role in Pat's arthritis. How much of a role does it play in others with this disease?

Multiple Sclerosis

Clinical and epidemiologic (health-related statistics among populations) data suggest that mercury from dental amalgam leaching into the body for many years may lead to multiple sclerosis later in mid-life.[174]

Multiple Sclerosis (MS) is described as an autoimmune (self-attacking), degenerative, inflammatory disease of the central nervous system. The disease process destroys the insulation on our "wires" (nerves), resulting in a short circuit. The cause is unknown. Rare in children, it is most often diagnosed between 20 and 40 years of age. There is no known cure.

The course of MS varies widely. There can be periods of dysfunction followed by periods of remission. Or, in a small percentage of cases, it can progress quickly and end in death within a few months. However, the average duration of MS is 30 years. Most MS patients can lead productive lives for many years.

The onset of MS can be very fast. As many as 40% of onsets happen within a few hours. Half the time, the first signs of MS are weakness and/or numbness in one or more limbs. Other symptoms can include difficulty in walking, double vision, involuntary eye movement, dizziness, vomiting and difficulty in urinating. It is common for those with MS to exhibit anger, depression and irritability.

There is no specific treatment that alters the eventual course of the disease.[175]

A 1994 study clearly demonstrates that mercury decreases nerve tissue's ability to produce actin and tubulin. Actin and tubulin are proteins found inside nerve cells and are necessary for proper nerve structure and function. Significantly, the study's results were based on mercury concentrations equivalent to that found in monkey brain only 28 days after amalgam was placed in the animal's teeth.[176] The question which arises from these findings is: Does mercury from amalgam in humans alter the structure and function of nerve cells resulting in nerve degeneration such as that seen in Multiple Sclerosis, Alzheimer's Disease and other degenerative nerve disorders?

I believe it is more than a coincidence that mercury intoxication and MS have nearly identical symptoms.

As early as 1940, a study demonstrated that four men who inhaled dust containing an organic mercury compound had initial symptoms including numbness and tingling of limbs, unsteadiness in gait, difficulty in performing fine motor tasks (buttoning a shirt), irritability and constricted visual fields.[177] Similar results have been found in other studies.[178, 179]

The mental health of MS patients with amalgam and MS patients with their amalgams removed was studied in 1992. The results are interesting. The group with amalgams showed significantly more depression, hostility, psychotism and obsessive-compulsive behavior than the group without amalgam. The group with amalgams reported 43% more mental health symptoms over the previous year than did the group without amalgam. It was concluded that the poorer mental health displayed by MS patients with amalgam may be linked with the mercury they ingest from their fillings. [180]

Another 1994 study completed at the Rocky Mountain Research Institute in Fort Collins, Colorado, found more significant evidence regarding the presence of mercury amalgams and MS. Scientists studied two groups of MS subjects, one which had amalgams removed and one which still had the fillings. The MS group with amalgams had a significantly lower red blood cell count and lower oxygen-carrying capacity than the group that had no mercury fillings. Also, the group with mercury fillings had worse kidney and thyroid measurements as well as lowered white blood cell counts and weaker immune system values. During the year of this study, the group with amalgams had 33.7% more MS symptom flare-ups than the amalgam-free group.

This same study researched and found a direct relationship between the prevalence of dental decay and MS. It is estimated that nearly 80% of all tooth decay is filled with mercury amalgam. The scientists studied the decay rates and MS rates in 47 countries, including the U.S. and Australia. The less decay reported, the less MS was found. The more decay reported, the more MS was found. The areas of highest decay rates were Northern Ireland and the Scottish islands of Orkney and Shetland. These are the same areas discovered to have the highest MS rate. Chinese residents of the U.S. were found to have a very low decay and MS rate.[181] Coincidences are adding up, aren't they? There are more . . .

Dental amalgam was first used as a filling in the U.S. in 1833. The lesions of MS were first described in 1838. The more widely amalgam was used, the more MS was seen.

In conclusion, the scientists remind us of interesting parallels. Mercury poisoning, called acrodynia, has multiple symptoms, including: weakness; moderate to severe pain in the arms and legs; redness and dry feeling of hands, feet and nose; irritability; sweating and irregular heart beat. In the late 1940s, it was thought by medical professionals that MS could be the adult form of acrodynia.[182]

I would suspect that most people with MS certainly would not want to be exposed to any material that has been shown to cause MS-like symptoms, such as amalgam fillings. Maybe tooth decay and MS have a common cause unrelated to mercury. But it seems logical to investigate these strong correlations first.

A case history

I have had patients with varying degrees of MS. Some have requested that the mercury be removed from their mouths and they have reported slight to significant improvements in their symptoms. Those with less advanced symptoms, younger patients and patients who ate well and maintained a positive attitude progressed further and faster. Older patients, those with medical or attitudinal challenges and those who had MS for a long time progressed more slowly and with less dramatic results.

One patient I had was a healthy young man in his early 20s, close to 200 pounds and about six feet tall. He was in the U.S. military, soon to be stationed in Germany. He had come to me as a patient because he had family near my office. I gave him an examination and a cleaning. He needed a number of fillings and decided to have the military dentist do them, as it would be free. Nothing in his health history indicated any medical problems. By all measures, he seemed very healthy. Several mercury amalgams had been in his mouth for many years.

As is often the case in military service, he had to have all his dentistry completed before he went to Germany. So a military dentist removed the decay and placed mercury fillings in his teeth.

The first signs of MS began while he was in Europe. He had trouble walking and lost weight. The symptoms worsened. He was diagnosed with MS and given a medical discharge. He knew I was a health-centered, mercury-free dentist and decided to have all his mercury amalgams removed.

When I saw him, I was shocked. He wobbled through my office door, barely able to walk. His weight had decreased by 50 pounds and he looked very, very ill. My heart felt heavy to see this once healthy young man in such a weakened condition. With a great deal of effort, he sat down in the chair and revealed to me his story. I could barely understand his words because his speech was so slurred. (Speech difficulties are common in MS.)

I removed his mercury amalgams. After his last removal visit, I did not see him for some time. Then one day about six months later, he walked in the office with a steady happy gait and shook my hand. He told me in a clear voice he had gained back 50 pounds and had plans to be married soon. He looked and acted like a new man.

He is now married and is ecstatic to be a father. He has not recovered completely, but the improvement has been dramatic.

So what might have caused this young man's "MS"? Let me give a parallel example and then explain. After taking a particular drug such as penicillin several times, the body can develop what is called a hypersensitivity to it. In other words, the body can develop an allergy or a sensitivity to a substance through repeated contact. The body may eventually say, "enough is enough" and no longer be able to tolerate the substance.

The body can react that way to mercury. New amalgam emits a lot more mercury than old amalgam. My young patient's new fillings gave him an increased dose of mercury. That might have been the final drop of water that spilled the whole cup. It may have been his triggering dose. Stories such as his must not be ignored or dismissed as coincidence.

Great medical and scientific discoveries have been and will continue to be made by observation. Penicillin, one of this century's most important developments, was discovered by "accident" during a bacterial culture experiment. In 1928, Sir Alexander Fleming noticed a green patch of mold growing on one of his culture dishes. There was a clear ring of no bacterial growth all around the mold. Through more experiments, he found out that this mold produced a substance we now call penicillin. His life was saved by his own discovery when he contracted pneumonia.[183] If he had ignored the observation, or dismissed it, who knows when we may have had penicillin available to save lives?

Other heavy metals besides mercury, such as lead and cadmium, also seem to cause symptoms like those of multiple sclerosis. Studies must be conducted to find out why people across the U.S. with MS seem to improve when mercury is removed from their teeth. If it is possible, let us find a cause for disorders such as MS. If we find a cause, we can find a method of prevention and maybe we can find a way to stop the further progression of such devastating diseases.

Cancer

Close to a million new cancer cases are diagnosed each year in the U.S. Our immune system protects us from cancer. Because exposure to mercury has been demonstrated to suppress the immune system, mercury may increase the chance of getting cancer.

Links between mercury-containing fungicides and leukemia (cancer of the blood cells) in farmers as well as their cattle were noted in 1987.[184]

Chapter 4

If mercury is linked to leukemia in any way, should it be allowed in fillings? And, because mercury lowers the immune system's ability to fight disease and sickness, no one is getting healthier by breathing mercury from dental fillings. This is especially true for people who already have a serious disease. Certainly someone with cancer should avoid ingesting mercury. No matter what causes the disease, mercury exposure may make it worse.

AIDS (HIV infection)

AIDS is thought by most researchers to be caused by a virus called the human immunodeficiency virus (HIV). But some highly respected researchers and physicians disagree. There are some recent indications that AIDS can be transmitted without the HIV virus, which may be just a tag-along.[185,186] However, most scientists believe the virus attaches itself to a type of T cell, the T4 specifically, destroying the cell and causing progressive suppression of the immune system.

Is it realistic to expect that removal of mercury amalgams may slow the progression of AIDS? I believe the answer is yes. AIDS is a disease of the immune system, which mercury can suppress in multiple ways. It makes sense that if mercury exposure was removed as a factor in AIDS that the patient could only benefit.

However, the process of removing amalgam exposes the patient to a temporary high concentration of mercury vapor. It is extremely important, therefore, for the patient to be fully protected while the removal takes place. (see "Amalgam replacement for health-challenged people," page 224). It is also advisable for the dentist and patient to work closely with a physician. It may even be advisable not to attempt such a procedure at all on extremely sick patients. Obviously, the earlier in the disease process that amalgams are removed, the longer one may benefit.

Dr. Hardy's Theory on Autoimmune Diseases

Modern medicine has identified a number of diseases as autoimmune. The prefix "auto" means "self" and in an autoimmune disease the body seems to destroy its own tissue -- its own self -- for no reason at all.

I believe that there is no such thing as an autoimmune disease.

There are many diseases currently thought of as being autoimmune. They include rheumatoid arthritis, multiple sclerosis, Grave's disease, systemic Lupus erythematosis, Reiter's syndrome, glomerulonephritis, hemolytic anemia, myasthenia gravis, insulin-dependent diabetes mellitus and chronic thyroiditis.[187]

Scientists scratch their heads and possibly other body parts as they look under the microscope and watch what appears to be normal tissue being destroyed by the immune system's armies.

I believe that there are no autoimmune diseases because I don't believe normal tissue is being attacked in these illnesses. I believe the attacked tissue only appears normal and has been altered at the atomic level. For instance, an atom may have been added or removed from a molecule of tissue. The body then correctly recognizes this changed tissue as foreign and sets it under siege. The scientists, however, don't realize the tissue has been altered, because today's microscopes aren't strong enough to see these atomic changes. So to the researchers, the body appears to be destroying normal tissue for no reason.

I feel that autoimmune disorders are, in reality, atomic disorders. When the molecular structure, or normal three dimensional shape of certain body molecules is distorted by the abnormal addition or removal of atoms, the immune system recognizes this and attempts to destroy the molecule. In some cases, the abnormal addition or removal may be more than one atom; it may be an entire added or removed molecule. The molecule may still be unidentifiable using the current microscopes.

It may be within each specific structural change that the true cause(s) for each specific autoimmune disorder may be discovered.

Drop out of the experiment

Dose determines the severity of poisoning. How much does it take to make you sick? How long can you take low-level mercury exposure before illness arrives? Why would anybody want to be the research subject to find out? Because these and other important questions remain unanswered, everyone with amalgam in their mouth is part of the experiment. The good news is that you can drop out of the experiment. Use safer, stronger and better-looking mercury-free fillings on the market now. The cost to replace fillings is not drastic. Now is the time for consumers to stand up and tell dental professionals that they refuse to have mercury amalgam in their mouths.

MUSCULOSKELETAL

Lou Gehrig's disease (ALS)

The symptoms of Lou Gehrig's disease, otherwise known as amyotophic lateral sclerosis (ALS), include muscular weakness, especially in the hands or feet, cramping and twitching. Later, speech and swallowing difficulties ensue. [188]

Two studies report of mercury intoxication resembling ALS:

In the first, two workers exposed to high concentrations of inorganic mercury particles had muscular pain in the lower back and extremities, severe burning sensations in the lower legs and feet and muscle cramping and twitching. The author noted that the symptoms were reminiscent of ALS.[189] Unlike ALS, though, all symptoms subsided three months after the exposure to the mercury particles ended.

The second report tells of a 54-year-old man having symptoms simulating ALS after a brief but intense exposure to mercury vapor. This apparently happened three months after he had spent two days salvaging mercury from thermometers. He developed muscle twitching, fatigue, unsteadiness in his handwriting, tingling, numb sensations in his hands and feet and severe constipation. In six weeks, he lost more than 20 pounds. He was forced to quit his job due to fatigue.

Five-and-a-half months after the exposure to the mercury vapor, his symptoms had disappeared and he began to gain weight. He returned to his job and was free of symptoms two-and-one-half years later. It was felt that his symptoms went away and stayed away because he was no longer exposed to mercury vapor. The report's authors said that mercury intoxication must be considered in cases of unexplained muscle and nerve disorders as well as psychiatric symptoms such as depression and confusion.[190]

NEUROLOGIC/ PSYCHOLOGIC

The most critical target organ of mercury vapor or organic mercury exposure is universally recognized to be our central nervous system. Our central nervous system (CNS) includes our brain and spinal cord, along with all the nerves and organs that control voluntary and involuntary acts. The parts of our brain that govern consciousness and mental activities are part of our CNS.[191] Anything that adversely affects our CNS affects our outlook on life. Therefore, breathing mercury vapor can effect our ability to react physically, mentally and emotionally in our day to day living.

Short-term, intermediate and long-term exposure to mercury elicit similar nerve problems. The signs and symptoms increase and may become permanent as mercury exposure lengthens or its concentration rises.[192] The type of exposure to mercury vapor

123

from amalgams is termed chronic or long-term exposure. So, even though the level of mercury vapor from amalgams may be low, it may elicit nerve problems in the long term due to accumulation.

There are so many negative effects from mercury exposure on the nervous system that I will list them first. Then I'll discuss a few representative signs and symptoms.

Neurologic symptoms of mercury exposure include:

Abnormal brain wave patterns (EEG)
Anxiety
Attention deficit disorder (ADD)
Cerebral Palsy
Depression
Difficulty walking
Drowsiness
Fits of anger
Hallucinations (in severe poisoning)
Headaches
Insomnia
Irritability
Loss of self control
Loss of intellect
Loss of memory
Loss of self-confidence
Manic depression
Nervousness
Speech difficulties
Tremors
Shyness or timidity
Visual disturbances [193,194,195,196]

It truly is amazing how many different signs of mercury poisoning there are. That is the major reason it is so difficult to diagnose. It can look like so many different illnesses. The numerous faces of mercury poisoning reveal the depths of mercury's danger. It is the master of disguise.

The most delicate system

The nervous system, in all probability, is the most delicate system when it comes to mercury toxicity. Other body systems may be able to repair mercury's damage, while nervous system damage may remain forever.

Most studies have shown that muscle-related problems, such as weakness and mild tremor, were reversible following the removal of the mercury source. However, mental impairments, especially memory problems, may be permanent due to irreversible CNS damage.[197,198]

Long-term, low-level mercury vapor exposure -- what one receives from amalgam -- affects the peripheral nervous system. This system includes all nerves outside the brain and spinal cord. There is a high prevalence of peripheral nerve problems among dentists. These include slower muscle movements and nerve reaction times.

Proper muscle movement and nerve reaction times are essential in performing and coordinating manual skills. I don't have to tell you how important these skills are to a dentist, and, all dentists who handle and place amalgam are exposed to mercury vapor daily. Amalgam-exposed dentists have reported stress, vision problems, decreased feelings in the legs and increasing loss of ability to perform dental skills.[199,200,201]

These dentists are being poisoned by the very same amalgam the ADA says is safe. Your dentist may be poisoned. I am upset that so many intelligent and hard-working dental professionals are kept in the dark about mercury's toxic effects. Dental schools, if they address it at all, only skim the subject and ADA spokespersons carefully select sources in favor of using mercury.

I believe that if dentists were given all the facts, most would choose not to work with amalgam. I also believe that the majority of dentists are conscientious and devoted. To have them unknowingly exposed to such a poison is tragic.

I have chosen to be mercury-free. I and my staff benefit by having a healthier work place, and my patients benefit directly and indirectly as a result.

Two dentists, a father and son poisoning

The following story was reported in the *Journal of the American Dental Association* (JADA).

In Utah, a father and son, both dentists, shared an office building. The two developed worsening symptoms over a very long time. Heavy fatigue engulfed the father along with a shooting pain in his neck. His right hand became swollen, painful and felt hot. Later symptoms included numbness and an open ulcer on his left leg. It was the same leg which was under the machine that mixed the mercury filling material before it was placed in a patient's mouth.

The son developed a depressing fatigue along with sudden numbness in his toes and feet. Increasingly poor reflexes in his feet, knees and legs caused difficulty in walking. A strong metallic taste was in his mouth. His head shook and his neck felt like it was being electrically shocked when he bent his head forward.

A mercury vapor testing device was brought to the office. Mercury vapor levels were so high in some office areas that the device was unable to measure them. Both dentists used amalgam-mixing machines that spilled mercury onto the countertop. The mercury then fell on the floors, greatly increasing the contamination. They also used the same ventilation system, so the mercury vapor was distributed throughout the building. Several measures to reduce the mercury vapor were taken, but the use of mercury amalgam by both dentists continued.

Finally, according to the article, the mercury contamination was cleared up, but the ulcer on the father's leg did not heal for a year. The son continued to have numbness in his legs and feet and his reflexes did not fully return to normal even though he took medication.[202]

If I were to go through what either of these dentists had been through, I would never go back into that building or any other where mercury had been or was being used. And I surely would not continue to work with the same dangerous material that caused the problems in the first place. This is beyond my comprehension! How many dentists suffer from similar symptoms and have no idea that mercury from dental amalgam is the cause? How confident can you be that mercury vapor levels are safe in your dentist's office? Safe levels of poison for one person may be disease-causing for another. If mercury amalgam is used in the office, there is mercury vapor present. Remember, mercury vapor has no smell and cannot be detected by human senses. The highest concentrations of mercury vapor come from mixing and placing new amalgam. A mercury-free office would have no new amalgam. It would tend to have more safeguards against mercury exposure during amalgam removal than an office that felt amalgam was safe.

Alzheimer's disease

Alzheimer's disease is characterized by progressive, irreversible loss of memory and intellectual ability as well as speech and walking disturbances, apathy and disorientation. It results from atrophy (decreasing size) of parts of the brain. Its exact cause is not yet clear. Most cases start between age 40 and 60 and may take anywhere from months to years to fully progress to complete loss of intellectual function.[203]

Autopsy studies of Alzheimer's victims have revealed high levels of mercury in the brains.[204,205,206] And an animal study has demonstrated that mercury caused brain damage similar to that seen in

127

Alzheimer's.[207]

One man underwent a reversal of his disease. A CAT scan of his brain on June 11, 1983, allegedly confirmed a diagnosis of Alzheimer's disease. Three doctors diagnosed him identically. He had been given seven years to live, marked by his progressive deterioration.

Deciding not to accept the diagnosis as irreversible and terminal, he studied and learned as much as possible about Alzheimer's. He ate wholesome foods, avoided foods and chemicals to which he was allergic, took vitamin and mineral supplements and had his amalgam fillings removed. Less than a year after the amalgams were removed, on April 4, 1987, a second CAT scan was done. The Alzheimer's had allegedly reversed itself, something medical textbooks say is not possible. Several specialists all confirmed that the Alzheimer's was reversed. He credited his recovery in large measure to the removal of his amalgam fillings.[208]

Anxiety

I saw a patient of mine recently, Carolyn, who told me something exciting. She had gotten off of a drug she had been on for ten years. It was an anti-anxiety drug. The only change in her life was the removal of her mercury amalgam fillings. She attributed her being able to stop the drug to the removal of amalgams.

I asked if she realized that anxiety was one of the first symptoms to arise from mercury exposure. She said no. I told her about the Mad Hatter syndrome which was discovered in the hat making industry in the 1800s. Mercury was used to shape hats and the exposed hatters became mad. The madness ranged from anxiety to mood swings to depression to severe personality changes and abnormal thought processes (see "The Mad Hatters", page131).

It is quite possible that Carolyn's anxiety, at least in part, was caused by exposure to mercury from her amalgams.

Nine medical lab technicians were treated for irritability, shyness, fatigue, headaches, nightmares, anxiety, tension, depression and forgetfulness. They had difficulty concentrating and focusing. Some of the women complaining were thought by their physicians to be neurotic. But an investigation of their workplace (cardiac laboratories) discovered significant levels of mercury in the atmosphere.[209] Who else is dismissed as neurotic but really has mercury toxicity?

Attention Deficit Disorder (ADD)

So many children are increasingly diagnosed with attention deficit disorders (ADD) and just put on drugs. Some are considered bright but hyperactive. Putting a child on strong drugs is often done with mixed feelings, but what else can help? Let's look at a possible link between ADD and mercury exposure.

By far, the most common filling used in children and adults is mercury amalgam. What does ADD look like in children and adult patients? Neuroses, depression, anxiety, irritability, shyness, forgetfulness, tension, headaches, nightmares and fatigue. These are all signs of mercury poisoning.

How many cases of learning disorders, ADD and depression in our school-aged children may be traced to their teeth?

Cerebral Palsy(see Birth Defects page 93)

Depression/fits of anger

In a study of mental patients' blood, elevated levels of mercury were found in a number of cases, especially those with depression and severe mental disturbances.[210]

This has huge significance for the mental health profession. If mercury exposure is implicated in depression and severe mental disturbances, what role does dental amalgam play in mental illness? It has been estimated that 100 million people in the U.S. alone have mercury amalgams. Could the presence of amalgam-released mercury vapor in mentally ill patients worsen their illness?

Would some disturbed patients be productive without their amalgams? How much depression is caused by amalgam? How much violent behavior may be caused by mercury from amalgam? Is violence made worse by mercury exposure? How much crime may be attributed to mercury from amalgam? Could we notice a reduction in violent tendencies if we remove amalgams in convicts? Could we reduce crime if everyone's teeth became mercury-free? Would the current level of violence show a decline?

Mental disturbances, including depression and fits of anger, can give birth to violent behavior or crime. Mood swings and fits of anger are common psychiatric signs of mercury poisoning. Sometimes the behavior is directed inward as in suicide (see "suicide," page 133). Other times, it may be directed outward. Our society does not need any assistance increasing the crime rate, the suicide rate or the mental illness rate.

A good step away from these woes would be to remove the single largest source of mercury exposure to the public: dental amalgam. Because of the huge potential for harm to so many people, I support a complete ban on amalgam fillings.

Drowsiness

In a 1989 study, workers exposed to low levels of inorganic mercury in the air demonstrated an increase in sleep disorders and memory disturbances.[211]

Drowsiness often plagues people with chronic fatigue syndrome. A symptom of mercury poisoning is chronic fatigue. A fair number of accidents in cars, boats, planes and trains can be traced to fatigue and drowsiness. How much does the mercury coming off amalgams contribute to accident-causing drowsiness?

The Mad Hatters

Nearly everyone who has read or seen Alice's adventures beyond the looking glass remembers the Mad Hatter's tea party. The hatter was lovable one moment and hateful the next. He would be genteel, then suddenly rude. He didn't make much sense and his emotions seemed to be on the Coney Island roller coaster. He was, in fact, poisoned by mercury. The mad hatters were real people.

The Mad Hatter in "Alice in Wonderland" was a caricature of a very serious workplace problem in the 1800s. The hat industry used a mixture of mercury and nitric acid to treat fur to make felt hats.[212] The hatters breathed the poisonous mercury all day at work and suffered brain damage leading to insanity, hence the phrase "mad as a hatter."

According to Webster's unabridged dictionary, "mad as a hatter" means completely crazy. In fact, the Occupational Safety and Health Administration states that the fur and felt hat industries in the U.S. were a major source of mercury poisoning until about 1940 when a less poisonous chemical replaced mercury.[213] I want to know how long the dental industry will take to learn what the fur and felt hat industry knew in 1940: mercury is poisonous.

What has the medical profession done to study mercury's role in certain psychological diseases? In particular, what has the medical or dental profession done to study the role chronic mercury exposure from dental amalgam plays in the psychological health of the estimated 100 million Americans who have them? To date, there are no tests that determine preclinical stages or diseases arising from mercury vapor exposure on organ systems such as the central nervous system.[214] The challenge for the medical, dental and psychological professions is to determine mercury's role in mental disorders.

Panic Disorder (see Anxiety pg. 128)

Chapter 4

Personality Disturbances

I gave a presentation to a Kiwanis group on February 5, 1993. One of the guests happened to be a highly respected police officer responsible for the arrest of serial murderer Ted Bundy. After I had talked for a while, he raised his hand and said, "I've been listening to you describe how low-level exposure to mercury vapor can cause subtle personality changes and I'd like to tell you of what happened to me. Until now, I thought it was just a coincidence. When I turned 40, I felt better than I had in years. I thought it was just because I had made it to 40, but I just had all my fillings taken out and replaced with caps. It makes me wonder how much my fillings may have been affecting me. My former wife noticed such a change in my personality that she said, 'You're so nice now. If you had been that nice when we were together, we'd still be married.'"

I can't help but get upset when I realize that two people who once loved each other enough to marry may have been torn apart by a personality change brought on slowly by mercury leaching from fillings. The most subtle effects of low-level chronic mercury poisoning are usually the first to show. They are related to personality: mood swings, depression, anxiety, irritability and fits of anger.

How many children's lives may be altered by divorce or discontent due to the subtle mercury exposure their parents get each day from dental fillings? How many dysfunctional children grow up to be dysfunctional parents, in part, because of mercury vapor exposure? What about violence in the home? Does mercury play a role? How many crimes may be committed because an otherwise calm individual's personality is warped and twisted by this psychological poison?

Subtle effects

I am very concerned about mercury's subtle effects, its more obscure effects. Mercury fillings give off low levels of mercury 24 hours a day, accumulating slowly over time. Because the symptoms usually come on gradually, they often go unnoticed for a long while. Symptoms can sneak up quietly, slowly.

How many people would attribute the stiffness in their joints, painful colitis, headaches, gum disease, or the asthma to the mercury fillings they've had in their mouth for 20 years? Indeed, how many physicians even know "silver" fillings contain 50% to 70% mercury? How many physicians would consider mercury as a possible source for these widely varying symptoms, even if they did know? Very few physicians diagnose mood swings, depression, anxiety, short-term memory loss, fits of anger, headaches, colitis or joint pain as chronic mercury poisoning, even though the quantity of scientific literature describing these symptoms is substantial. Often, the patients with psychological symptoms end up being referred to psychiatrists, psychologists and/or counselors.

The subtle effects of mercury mimic other disorders and diseases. Diagnosis in some cases is difficult. So, wouldn't it be prudent and preventative if amalgams were eliminated from the realm of suspects altogether?

Suicide

It is commonly known that dentists have the highest suicide rate of any profession.[215] My explanation lies in what I see as the obvious: Dentists are exposed to far more mercury daily than any other profession. It has been estimated by the ADA that 75% of all tooth restorations are mercury amalgams. I know of no other profession that uses mercury on a daily basis at all, let alone for so much of their daily routine. Not only are dentists exposed from the amalgam they place in the mouth, but also from any drop of mercury or scrap of amalgam that has fallen to the floor or that sits on the table next to the patient. There may be mercury vaporizing today that was spilled in the office ten years ago! There is absolutely no way human senses can detect mercury vapor. Until symptoms begin to show, there is no way to tell what harm may be done.

Recall that mercury vapor exposure can bring on the Mad Hatter syndrome: mood swings, anxiety, depression, irritability and fits of anger. I see no major reason for the high rate of suicide among dentists other than mercury exposure. We earn good wages, are usually self-employed, work good hours and are well-respected members of the medical profession. Dentistry can't be more stressful than anesthesiology, surgery or cancer treatment. Yet the professionals dealing with these severe medical situations apparently handle their stress better than dentists. The difference, I believe, lies in mercury exposure.

My staff and I take many precautions during the removal of mercury amalgams. We wear special mercury-absorbing masks, use ionizing air filtration combined with powdered sulfur and, at night, ozonate the office air. But I still feel more moody and tired when I've removed a lot of amalgam from patients' mouths. I feel less so when I've had a busy day but with no amalgam removal. And when I go on vacation, I notice a big difference in my level of composure. Surely some of this inner peace comes from the vacation itself, but I'm just as sure that some comes from being away from any source of mercury, however slight. I notice a difference in myself and my wife does, too.

Teen suicide

Teen suicide is a major problem today. I have mentioned that most amalgam fillings placed in children are done between ages 9 and 15. These young, rapidly-developing bodies can be hit with several fillings at once, vaporizing mercury 24 hours a day. If dentists have the highest suicide rate of any profession because of exposure to mercury from amalgam, I wonder what role dental amalgam may have in teen suicide?

OCULAR / DERMAL
(eye and skin)

Humans exposed to mercury vapor have developed diffuse (scattered) red and itchy skin rashes.[216,217] Inorganic mercury exposure in humans has been reported to cause itchy measle-like spots, fever, mouth inflammation and a red rash over the face and body.[218]

Mercury's effects on the eyes include redness, burning and inflammation of the mucous membranes lining the eyelids. People exposed to a low concentration of mercury have had double vision and a greyish-brown or yellow haze on the outer surface of their eyes.[219,220,221]

Mild to severe eye irritations were noticed in a large number of people using contact lens saline solutions that contained the preservative, thimerosal. (Thimerosal is the chemical name for the mercury compound known as Merthiolate.)With increased use of mercury preservatives in the saline solutions, the number of eye irritations grew. In 1983, up to 50% of contact lens wearers in the United States were affected.[222,223] The saline manufacturers realized something had to be done and began making saline solutions for "sensitive eyes." When they used the phrase "for sensitive eyes" it really meant "for eyes sensitive to mercury preservatives." How many people realized that the problems they were experiencing with their contact lenses were from mercury? (see "Merthiolate in my eyes", page 164)

ORAL CAVITY (mouth)

Nausea, vomiting and inflammation of the mouth are commonly-found symptoms in mercury vapor exposure.[224] Other symptoms affecting the mouth created by exposure to mercury include:

Bleeding gums
Bone loss
Burning sensation of the mouth or throat

Excessive salivation
Foul breath
Loosening of teeth
Leukoplakia (white patches)
Metallic taste
Stomatitis (inflammation of the mouth)
Tissue pigmentation
Ulceration of the gums, palate and tongue.

Gum disease (Periodontitis): the most prevalent disease in America

I was taught in dental school that the most common disease in America is gum disease. Research shows that the very same symptoms which describe gum disease can be produced by mercury exposure.

It has been estimated that 85 percent of adults over 35 have periodontal disease.[225] "Perio" means surrounding and "dontal" means pertaining to the teeth; hence periodontal disease is the disease of the structures surrounding teeth. It is so common that there is a dental specialty just for gum disease called periodontics.

Gum disease is a silent disease. There are usually few if any warning signs. Often, only bleeding gums and bad breath can alert a person that he or she may have gum disease. I find that once most people understand what causes gum disease, they want to stop it. Gum disease (periodontitis) is probably the easiest disease to stop. Let me explain what it is.

Mouth bacteria are avid construction workers, constantly building "houses" called plaque on the teeth. The bacteria prefer to build in areas that do not have food sliding over the surface each time a meal goes through, so most plaque ends up between the teeth. Within 24 hours their houses begin to harden into what is called calculus. Once the houses harden, flossing and brushing won't knock them off. Only a professional cleaning with the proper instruments will clean the teeth.

Each day, another floor is added to the hardened houses. In this way, the bacteria build multistory condos on the teeth. There are no bathrooms in these condos so all the waste products from the millions, often billions of bacteria living in the calculus condos ooze out into the gums. This flow of waste creates inflamed gums, a condition called gingivitis. The body is trying to fight the waste when gums get red and puffy.

As the calculus condos get bigger and more bacteria move in, more waste flows into the gums. This population explosion causes more severe inflammation and deepens the gum pockets (naturally occurring collars of gum around the neck of each tooth) by actually destroying the bone around the tooth. If the body can't remove the source of the infection, eventually it moves the bone and gums away. The vicious cycle has begun. Once the gum pockets deepen, even more condos can be built farther down the tooth's root surface. The deeper and lower the condos, the harder for the body to fight the waste flow, so more and more bone around the teeth is destroyed.

Gum disease is an infection, so it robs the immune system of some of the defensive capabilities that it would normally use to fight colds, flu, cancer, AIDS, or any other medical challenge.

Gum disease can eventually end in tooth loss.

Tooth loss is documented in the scientific literature to also be a symptom of mercury exposure. As early as the 1700s, mercury miners' teeth were known to have fallen out.[226]

A 1990 study reported that patients hypersensitive to mercury (determined by a patch test) had stomatitis (inflammation of the mouth) wherever amalgams touched. This inflammation disappeared when amalgams were removed, but remained in the patient who decided against removal.[227] Bleeding gums and stomatitis were reported as common symptoms in several other studies as well.[228,229,230,231,232,233]

As a dentist, the last thing I want to do is increase the prevalence of any mouth disorders, especially periodontal disease. No study that I am aware of has looked at how the effects of low mercury doses over a lifetime of amalgam fillings correlate to the occurrence of gum disease. Why is that, especially when a large body of well-respected research demonstrates that the very same symptoms found in periodontal disease may be produced by mercury exposure? How many periodontists realize this similarity and see certain cases improve with amalgam removal? Some periodontists have referred cases to me for mercury amalgam removal. The patients and doctors have been pleased with the results. Amalgam should not be used in patients with gum disease.

RENAL (kidney)

A dental assistant died of kidney failure as a result of exposure to mercury vapor from the dental amalgam with which she worked.[234] I'm sure that if the assistant were able to say something about mercury use in dentistry, it would be to ban it forever. I will speak for her. How many other dental assistants have died from kidney failure but were not diagnosed properly nor written up in the scientific literature? How many more may die before amalgam is banned?

In an important study done in Canada, six sheep received 12 amalgam fillings. Two sheep received the same number of mercury-free fillings. The sheep with amalgam steadily lost kidney function. Within two months, up to 80% of their kidney function was gone. But the sheep that received the mercury-free fillings had no decrease in kidney function.[235] A 1990 study on mercury distribution from dental amalgam in monkey tissues repeated and confirmed the results found in sheep.[236]

The kidney is one of the major targets for mercury accumulation. Several degenerative changes can occur there following exposure to mercury vapor. Since kidneys have an enormously high capacity to concentrate mercury, symptoms can range from increased protein or blood in the urine to complete kidney failure.[237,238] Such damage may or may not be accompanied by an elevation of mercury found in the urine. This is important because some testing relies on urine mercury levels to determine exposure, and it has been found to be unreliable for determining mercury exposure.

It has been suggested that kidney dysfunction caused by mercury vapor might result from an autoimmune mechanism[239] (see Dr. Hardy's Theory on Autoimmune Diseases, page 121). In autoimmune disease, you may remember the body appears to attack seemingly normal tissue. Autoimmune dysfunction of the kidney caused by mercury vapor may fit the same theory I proposed for mercury-induced rheumatoid arthritis, also considered an autoimmune disease.

A friend of mine happens to be a dialysis nurse. I've learned a lot from her about kidneys. She said that once kidney tissue has lost its ability to function, it has almost always lost it forever. Kidneys are so proficient at filtering out waste and maintaining proper salt and pH balances, that a person can live on only 10% functioning of just one kidney. But, once someone is on dialysis, it usually is permanent. Only a donor kidney would be able to get a person off regular dialysis. And the waiting list for kidney recipients is extremely long. I have known several patients who have been on the waiting list for years, with no real prospects for a transplant in the near future.

Ironically, if mercury poisoning is the cause of a patient's kidney failure and the resultant dialysis, it cannot be removed by dialysis. Mercury is not listed among the dialyzable toxic substances.[240] The mercury would have to be removed by some other method.

Kidney problems caused by mercury poisoning are usually treated by what is called chelation therapy with BAL or Penicillamine. BAL is a sulfur-containing compound. Mercury is strongly attracted to sulfur. BAL's effectiveness may be due, in large part, to the presence of sulfur. Penicillamine is not only used for mercury poisoning, but also for treating rheumatoid arthritis and lead poisoning.[241]

We all have heard of the horrors of lead poisoning. Well, mercury is lead's dangerous twin. It is more poisonous than lead because it can enter the body more easily and in more forms. And mercury poisoning causes identical symptoms. Even the treatment for lead and mercury poisoning is the same.

Autopsy studies in California and Sweden have shown a direct correlation between the number of mercury amalgams and the quantity of mercury found in the brain and kidneys.[242] Isn't it disturbing to know that mercury found in your brain and kidneys can be directly related to the number of mercury fillings you may have?

RESPIRATORY
(lungs and airways)

The most efficient way to absorb mercury vapor is to breathe it. Mercury vapor is nearly 100% absorbed by lungs. As the vapor comes into contact with lung tissue, it can cause fluid retention, death of the lining of our airways and pneumonia. The mucus and fluid obstruction can result in emphysema, a rupture of the lung, chest pain, coughing, difficulty breathing and coughing blood.[243,244,245,246,247,248]

A fairly high number of people are mouth breathers, meaning they cannot breath through their nose very well or at all. If they have amalgams, each breath draws mercury vapor off the fillings into the lungs and directly into the bloodstream. If they chew gum, the friction heats up the amalgams, driving even more mercury off. Of course, if they have no amalgam fillings, they will not be inhaling mercury with every breath.

Asthma

Asthma is the most often diagnosed chronic illness in childhood and it can be devastating. Affected children are not able to play with the same intensity as their friends. Often they cannot play at all.

Running, exertion or excitement of any kind for some sufferers is enough to start an asthma attack.

Asthma is characterized by shortness of breath caused by airway constriction. Causes are listed as allergies, emotional stress, fatigue and unknown. Could mercury poisoning be removed from the unknown category and added as a cause of asthma?

Inhalation of mercury vapors can result in lung inflammation, airway inflammation, shortness of breath, lethargy or restlessness, abnormally rapid breathing, cough, partial or full collapsing of the lungs, emphysema, chest pain, bleeding and possibly death.[249,250,251,252] The mercury exposure one receives from amalgams is low-level and long-term. Is this level high enough or is the time of exposure long enough in some young people to create the symptoms of asthma? Each one of us is unique. So what may cause no signs for one child may cause illness in another.

On the basis of what is known about mercury's effects on the lungs and airways, mercury should be considered as a possible cause in some cases of asthma. How much does the mercury leaching off amalgams contribute to this disease especially in children, whose smaller bodies make them more susceptible to given quantities of toxins than adults? Mercury vapor coming off amalgams in a 200-pound adult will not have the same effect as it does on a 45-pound child.

I have noticed in my practice that before puberty about twice as many boys as girls need fillings due to decay. This may be due to better oral hygiene among girls. In adults, women catch up and the ratio is about even. Also before puberty, asthma attacks two times as many boys as girls. In adults, the rate is equal. Is this a coincidence? Or do the number of amalgam fillings correlate directly to the incidence of asthma?

C h a p t e r 4

BIOELECTROMAGNETICS (BEM)

The medicine of today is, for the most part, based on drug thera-py and surgery. I believe the medicine of the future will rely more heavily on electrical and magnetic therapies. They are less intrusive and have the potential for broad applications, less side effects and shorter recovery periods. After all, we are electrical and magnetic beings and science is just beginning to recognize the potential of this field of medicine, called bioelectromagnetics.

Every human being has his or her own set of natural electromag-netic fingerprints, and mercury fillings can influence them greatly. Every amalgam is a battery, a magnet and an antenna. When an amalgam is placed in a tooth, the natural electrical and magnetic fin-gerprint of the area changes. The more amalgam placed, the more the natural electromagnetic fields are changed. This might not be so bad if our teeth were in our feet, but they are next door to our brain. Anyone who's ever had a toothache knows how directly teeth are con-nected to the brain's pain center. Ouch!

Changing the natural electrical fingerprint so close to our brain may cause problems associated with our electrical systems. These may include numbness, paralysis, headaches, TMJ disorders (TMJ or jaw joint disorders include clicking, grinding, pain and inability to open wide), ringing in the ears, vision disturbances and changes in person-ality ranging from the mild to the severe.

Unexplained symptoms which I believe may be related to electri-cal disturbances in the mouth include:

Numbness or palsy in the face or neck
Hearing problems such as ringing in the ears
Vision disturbances
Headaches
Facial pain
Muscular problems, twitching or tension in face or neck

Teeth clenching or grinding
Emotional instability
Difficulty concentrating
Sensitivities in teeth

Composite resin, a superior filling material to amalgam, is electromagnetically neutral and therefore does not disturb the body's own natural electromagnetic fields.

What is BEM?

Bioelectromagnetics (BEM) is the name for a young science that integrates medicine, biology and physics. Bioelectromagnetics views disease and healing not in terms of surgery or pharmaceuticals, but through what are called electromagnetic (EM) fields.

Electromagnetic energy is all around us all the time. It is an ocean of invisible waves. It includes the Earth's own magnetic field, radio waves, TV waves, microwaves, radar and radar detectors, cellular phone waves, visible light, ultraviolet light, x-rays, gamma rays and cosmic rays.

Not only does each whole organism have an EM fingerprint, but each organ, indeed each cell, has its own EM fingerprint.

It has recently been discovered that at least some living cells contain magnetic crystals that respond to magnetic fields. Human brain cells and immune cells have been confirmed to have these crystals. This discovery enhances the theory that cells, organs and organisms may interact and communicate on the invisible level of electromagnetism.[253]

Research is being conducted on the harmful and beneficial effects of EM fields. The media has produced stories on the negative effects of EM fields from high tension overhead power lines, linking them to childhood leukemia. Now we are hearing bad news about video display terminals and cellular phones. On the positive side, BEM research is attempting to identify EM signals that may be used to boost the human immune system from outside the body. Other promising areas investigated for EM therapy are broken bones, osteoporosis, drug withdrawal, immune defects, AIDS and cancer. [254]

Why is BEM important in amalgams?

Human beings are BEM organisms. We have our own individual set of electrical, magnetic and chemical qualities. Similarities between us exist, but just as each of us has a different set of fingerprints, each of us has a unique EM fingerprint.

We are chemical, electrical and magnetic in our very nature. We see, hear, breathe, move, feel, think and communicate through electrical, magnetic and chemical impulses. When our electrical, magnetic and chemical systems are working properly, we, as organisms, are working properly.

Unfortunately, every mercury amalgam also has its own EM fingerprint. Each is a different size and shape and acts as a unique battery, magnet and antenna.

When a tooth is drilled to place a filling, the enamel is taken away. Under the enamel is dentin, a hard substance which has microscopic tubes running from the nerve chamber inside the tooth to the edge of the enamel. Inside these tubes are nerve fibers. This means that fillings can be placed in contact with nerve fibers. The filling, then, has a direct connection to the brain.

Headaches, TMJ symptoms, ringing in the ears and picking up radio stations have disappeared in many patients simply by removing the metallic amalgams. I believe that some headaches, TMJ symptoms and ringing in the ears may be caused by the change in normal electrical and magnetic fields brought on by the insertion of amalgam.

Two of my patients picked up radio stations so clearly they could tell me what was on the station at any given moment. (And neither was receiving a station they enjoyed!) In both cases, I removed the one filling I thought was receiving the station. I based my choice on research I had done on the electrical potentials of dental metals. Both patients were extremely grateful for the peace and quiet in their heads that followed. Sweet silence will never again be taken for granted.

One recent dramatic case of ringing in the ears stands out in my practice. Michael is 35. He had all his mercury fillings placed between nine and 12. By the age of 12 he suffered ringing in his ears 24 hours a day. The very day he had his last amalgam removed and replaced with composite resin, the ringing he had for 23 years was gone. Michael now feels he has a new life.

It may be that certain psychoses and mental disorders are caused by disturbances in normal EM fields. It may even be possible that certain arrangements of amalgams may cause mental disorders. Maybe just one amalgam can cause trouble. No one knows for sure. But there are 100 million people in the U.S. with amalgams to study. I'm sure there are some with mental and physical health challenges that would be thrilled to find a reason or even a partial reason for their troubles.

The great news is that the replacement fillings called composite resins are electrically neutral and do not disturb the natural EM fingerprint of the head and neck. Also because they are electrically neutral, they do not contribute to the corrosion of any other dental metals. As I have mentioned, fillings have a fairly direct connection to the tooth nerve, which is hard-wired to the brain. Therefore, choosing an electrically neutral filling is wise.

I have used composite resin fillings for nearly 14 years. In terms of color and wearability, they are the closest material to the natural tooth structure that the dental profession has. Their electrical qualities are similar to natural teeth. I have been very satisfied with my own composites, many of which have been in my molars for 14 years.

A computer runs best when all the parts are kept as close to original as possible. Normal voltage and current is essential. The same can be said of our bodies. Keep replacement parts as close to original as possible.

Chapter 4

CHILDREN'S VACCINES CONTAIN MERCURY!

Mercury compounds, no better than water, are still used as preservatives

I must discuss vaccines because many of them, made to be injected into the tiny bodies of infants, contain the master of disguise, mercury. Thimerosal, a compound using mercury, is used as a preservative in the vaccines. Thimerosal is the chemical name for what used to be called merthiolate, an over-the-counter antiseptic. Merthiolate was taken off the market after a death was reported to the FDA from it being dropped into ears for an ear infection.

Preservatives are supposed to kill or inhibit bacterial growth. As far back as 1950, a comprehensive study done on the ability of mercury compounds to kill or inhibit bacteria found that thimerosal was no better than water in protecting mice from potentially fatal streptococcal infection.[255] And the Advisory Review Panel on over-the-counter (OTC) mercury-containing drug products for the Food and Drug Administration classified thimerosal as "not generally recognized as safe and effective." The Panel concluded that "thimerosal is not safe for OTC topical use because of its potential for cell damage if applied to broken skin and its allergy potential."[256]

Well, I consider infants' skin that a needle has been pushed through to be broken skin. Why is a thimerosal-containing vaccine still being injected into babies and children? Maybe because nobody is questioning thimerosal's use in vaccines. Also, drug companies making vaccines have some of the most powerful lobbies in Washington, D.C.

DPT, combined diphtheria, tetanus and pertussis vaccine

According to at least one researcher, the DPT vaccination is the major cause of infant death, in the United States. It is also the most

146

preventable. The DPT shot contains formaldehyde (a known cancer-causing agent), aluminum and mercury. DPT is a combination of the vaccines for diphtheria, pertussis and tetanus.[257]

As many as 1 out of 200 vaccinated with the DPT series may experience severe reactions such as grand mal seizures and brain dysfunction. Eight times the normal death rate occurs in vaccinated children within three days after receiving DPT. The two peak ages at which Sudden Infant Death Syndrome occurs are at two months and four months. DPT's three primary doses are given at two months, four months and six months.[258] How much does mercury contribute to these grim statistics? Is thimerosal a preservative or a poison? If it is not effective as an over-the-counter antiseptic, how is it effective as a preservative? How much safer would the DPT shots be without mercury? Is mercury, injected into the infant, suppressing an already fragile and incomplete immune system? What role does mercury play in infant deaths from this vaccine?

Diphtheria

Among those who contract diphtheria, 50% have been properly vaccinated. In an official report on the toxoid vaccine, the FDA said the vaccine was not as effective as they had hoped and that permanent immunity was questionable.[259] Diphtheria vaccines contain mercury. What role does mercury play in the questionable immunity provided by this vaccine?

Hemophilus Influenza type B (GI)

The GI (Haemophilus b conjugate) vaccine, often mistakenly referred to as the meningitis vaccine, contains mercury. It is mandated in 44 states and is given to infants as young as 2 months old. Children who received the GI vaccine in Minnesota had a five times greater chance of contracting the disease than unvaccinated children.

(I am unclear as to whether the problem in Minnesota is due to the vaccine. If the vaccine was the cause, other states should also have the same statistics. It is possible that the only study conducted was in Minnesota). And 39 out of 55 children who contracted GI soon after vaccination developed meningitis.[260] What is mercury's role in vaccine-induced GI or meningitis?

Tetanus

Tetanus boosters can cause a transient lowering of T-lymphocyte blood count ratios. This can cause a temporary immune disorder in babies, lowering their ability to fight infection and to heal.[261]

Two types of tetanus vaccines are available. The tetanus antitoxin vaccine, an antidote for the tetanus poison, contains mercury. The tetanus toxoid vaccine, a deactivated form of the tetanus toxin, contains aluminum and mercury.

The diphtheria and tetanus vaccine for children contains mercury and aluminum, both human toxins and formaldehyde, a cancer-causing agent.

The diphtheria and tetanus for adults contains mercury and aluminum, but no formaldehyde.[262] It is not comforting to know that my young child's diphtheria and tetanus vaccine contains formaldehyde. I must ask again, why are these dangerous materials allowed in vaccines? What possible good can our body derive from aluminum, formaldehyde or mercury?

Other vaccines

Some vaccines such as the polio, measles, mumps and rubella vaccines do not contain mercury, but do contain antibiotics which may need reevaluation. Neomycin is toxic to the kidneys and may cause hearing problems.[263]

The live measles, live polio, measles, mumps and rubella

(MMR) and the measles and rubella vaccines all contain the antibiotic neomycin.[264] The measles vaccine has been linked to multiple sclerosis, Reye's Syndrome, Guillian-Barre' syndrome, blood-clotting problems and diabetes.[265]

The single largest cause of polio in the U.S. is from the live-virus polio vaccine, according to the Centers for Disease Control. As a matter of fact, every case of polio in the U.S. from 1980 through 1989 was caused by the vaccine. People are contagious for up to eight weeks after vaccination.[266] Are we giving polio to people who would not have had it without the vaccine? Would even more have gotten polio without the vaccine being used? The debate over whether polio vaccines are effective must center on these two questions.

The live oral polio vaccine contains two antibiotics: streptomycin and neomycin. The inactivated polio vaccine for injection contains formaldehyde (a cancer-causing agent) and alcohol.[267]

According to one source, one of the causes of Chronic Fatigue Syndrome (CFS) is the rubella vaccine. CFS symptoms are constant tiredness and lethargy to the point of drowsiness ranging from mild to severe. Headaches, joint pain, swollen lymph nodes, sore throat and low-grade fever are common. CFS may debilitate a person to where holding a job is impossible.

Joint pain, arthritis, peripheral nerve numbness, pain or paralysis are other side effects seen with the rubella vaccine. And if that were not enough, it seems that the rubella vaccine may be ineffective at best. One study revealed that 80% of army recruits contracted rubella (German measles) within four months of receiving the vaccine.[268] The rubella vaccine contains neomycin.[269]

These reports suggest a serious lack of oversight in rules governing the safety and effectiveness of vaccines. As a citizen and a parent, I want the FDA to require proof-of-safety studies done by independent researchers on all vaccines and their additives prior to use in the general population. Also, the studies need to address the specific reactions babies and children may experience with these products.

Vaccinations are supposed to prevent disease. The truth is that vaccines can sometimes cause the disease they were intended to prevent or cause undesirable side effects. Either should not be tolerated.

I support independent research that provides proof-of-safety of vaccines and their additives. I feel that the citizens of this country deserve the cleanest and safest vaccines science can make. To rest on the line that "we've always done it this way" is to shut the eyes and ears to dissent. Dissent, after all, is what made our country great. Let's all speak up for safer, cleaner vaccines.

In conclusion

As I see it, mercury amalgams cause 4 major problems:

1. They release chemically toxic mercury
2. They release immunologically toxic mercury
3. They create electrical and magnetic disturbances
4. They pollute our environment and lower our quality of life.

Mercury is the master element of disguise. It has no smell. It has no taste. It can enter the body as a vapor, a liquid or a solid. Once inside, it can change from one form to another. Because mercury is an element, it can not be broken down. Mercury, once released, is extremely difficult to contain. Although mercury atoms are smaller than microscopes can see, inside the body they can create a universe of trouble.

If mercury is the master of disguise, then amalgam fillings are the stage on which it acts and your body is the captive audience for its trickery and deception.

Hundreds of scientific articles attest to mercury's detrimental effects on virtually every system in the human body. Dental amalgam allows the 24-hour release of mercury into the body. The amount each amalgam releases may be small, but no one knows for certain at what level mercury may cause problems for any individual. We all have differing thresholds and abilities to withstand chemical, immunological and electrical insults.

Every amalgam also has its own electrical, magnetic and antenna characteristics. These may interfere with critical communication inside the human body, between human beings and between people and the environment. Examples of electrical interference symptoms include receiving radio stations on fillings, disturbances in hearing and personality changes.

In the U.S. we have sick houses, sick schools and sick buildings. We have processed foods containing a variety of chemical additives. We have mercury in our vaccinations for infants and children. We have mercury in 100 million people's fillings. And we have one of the highest violent crime rates on Earth.

We have stopped the use of the pesticide DDT. We can often clean up the sick buildings and the chemicals in food. We have stopped the use of the mercury-containing product Mercurochrome. And we can stop the use of mercury in vaccinations and dental fillings. These are not the only answers to violence, sickness and mental health problems, but they may be pieces of the puzzle. Let's put them in place.

Right now the demand for mercury amalgam keeps it the world's most used dental material. The consumer, by being unaware and accepting amalgam silently, feeds that demand. However, if the consumer decides against using such an antiquated toxic material, the demand will evaporate like water on a hot griddle. The four problems created by amalgam will simply go away when amalgam goes away. And, inside the body, mercury's universe of trouble will cease to exist.

Chapter 4

Our opinion matters

"Every revolution was first a thought in one man's mind and when the same thought occurs to another man, it is the key to that era. Every reform was once a private opinion and when it shall be a private opinion again, it will solve the problem of the age."
-Ralph Waldo Emerson

We are the power that creates history. Our opinions matter and are what ultimately decide issues. So, I believe it is important and necessary to express opinion. It is time to make a decision about the continued use of mercury.

George Washington had an opinion as to how this country could be created: for the people, by the people. I am of the opinion that we, the people, still have tremendous clout. We can make the dental profession change. We hold the power in our decisions. When we, as patients, refuse to accept mercury amalgam, dentists will use the superior filling material, composites. Composites have already been proven to be safer, stronger and more attractive than amalgam, without the mercury.

5

Chapter 5: Mercury On Earth

air, water

& soil

Mercury
On Earth

We are our environment

Environmental costs always come back to human costs. After all, we are, in a very real sense, our environment. We share billions of atoms with our air in every breath; billions more in every drop of liquid or scrap of food entering our bodies. We are the ultimate recycling machines.

I co-sponsored a talk given by Dr. Deepak Chopra in Orlando in October 1993. Dr. Chopra has written several best-selling books on the mind-body connection to health in which he describes how our environment lives in us as much as we live in our environment. I had dinner with him prior to the talk. He is a kind, humble and soft-spoken man with a wonderful sense of humor.

Every time I have heard him speak of how we share atoms with our environment, I feel connected to the earth the same way a rain drop is connected to a river, and the river to the oceans.

Dr. Chopra explains that atoms which used to be our heart, liver, kidneys, bones and brain are exhaled in each breath. Monthly all our skin is replaced, every five days we have a new stomach lining, in six weeks our liver is new, and in three months our skeleton. Though the arrangement of the atoms stays very much the same, every year we have 98% new atoms, making an entirely new body.[270]

Sharing our atoms with our environment gives us both health and disease. The more polluted our environment, the more our bodies will reflect this pollution. Conversely, the more polluted our bodies, the more we will spread it into our environment. We live in and through our environment as our environment lives in and through us.

The continual atomic interchange with the environment requires us to be wise with our choices. We must ask questions like, "What are the human risks of mercury in our environment?" "What is the largest source of mercury exposure for humans?" "What do we do to reduce our mercury exposure and, thereby, lead healthier, happier, more productive lives?"

This chapter will help you answer these questions and more. In it you will learn about the havoc that can follow when man puts mercury in the environment. You will learn some surprising places mercury may be found, such as your medicine cabinet and closet. You will learn of amalgams' possible effect in your dentist's office and on your dentist's body. You will learn the wonderful news that many countries are on their way toward banning amalgam and the terrible news that the U.S. is not.

Hopefully, after reading this chapter, you will conclude that it is wrong and unnecessary for dentists to be adding mercury to an already mercury-polluted environment and you will decide to request composite fillings from now on!

C h a p t e r   5

Mercury fillings are the largest source of mercury exposure in humans

The World Health Organization (WHO) studied mercury exposure to humans from air, water, food and amalgam fillings, and concluded that the largest source of exposure was, by far, dental amalgams. The WHO also concluded that there was no safe minimum dose of mercury. "Symptoms are known to occur, at least among some of the population, at every level of exposure."[271]

There is no safe level of mercury exposure. And we can remove the largest source of human mercury exposure by eliminating the use of mercury in dentistry. It is that simple.

Further support for the WHO conclusions came from four internationally recognized mercury researchers, Drs. Clarkson, Hursch, Nylander and Friberg who all concluded that mercury from dental amalgam was the largest source of inorganic mercury and mercury vapor exposure in the general population.[272]

It is clear amalgam presents the greatest mercury threat to human health. What about our larger body, our environment? What problems does mercury create there?

Mercury found in soil, water and air

This chapter discusses how dental mercury, found in our soil, water and air affects our lives. The problems and solutions of this mercury contamination will be covered. But first, let's understand why mercury cannot be broken down.

Mercury is forever

Pesticides and other industrial chemicals are often referred to as chemical compounds -- a mixture of elements. Dental amalgam, for instance, is a chemical mixture of mercury, silver, copper and tin or other trace metals. Chemical compounds can be broken down into the elements that make them up. For example, mercury amalgam breaks down into mercury, silver, copper and tin. Elements themselves -- like mercury -- cannot be broken down any further.

Once mercury is released, it can move or be moved from place to place, but it cannot be destroyed. In this respect, mercury is forever.

Mercury's use by man over the centuries has been laced with illness and death. Because of its toxicity, mercury has the dubious distinction of claiming two of the world's first environmental landmarks.

World's first occupational health standard, 1665

In 1665, the world's first occupational health standard was created for the mercury miners in what was once called Yugoslavia. Their workday was reduced from 14 to 6 hours because trembling, paralysis, malnutrition and premature deaths were occurring among the miners.[273]

World's first environmental lawsuit, in 1700s

What appears to be the world's first environmental lawsuit was filed in the early 1700s against a chemical factory making mercuric chloride. The suit claims the factory polluted the environment with mercury and caused an increase in the death rate in the immediate neighborhood.[274]

Mercury, lead's more dangerous twin

Almost everyone knows of lead's adverse health effects. Mental and physical damage can occur, ranging from lowered IQs to permanent physical handicaps. Mercury is more dense and deadly than lead. Lead even floats on liquid mercury. (As a matter of fact, lead is allowed in drinking water at concentrations 7.5 times that of mercury.)[274a] Mercury poisoning has symptoms identical to lead poisoning, but mercury is a liquid at room temperature, unlike lead. Being a liquid, mercury evaporates at normal temperatures, poisoning the air, while lead, being a solid, does not. Until lead melts, one cannot breathe its vapors. Mercury melts at -40 degrees Celsius or -129.6 degrees Fahrenheit. Lead doesn't liquefy or melt until it reaches 327.4 degrees Celsius or 621.3 degrees Fahrenheit.[275]

If you leave water in a pot at room temperature, it eventually evaporates (turns into vapor). Mercury does the same. Lead, because it remains solid, does not. This is why mercury is more dangerous than lead. Mercury vapor -- the main exposure from mercury fillings -- allows mercury great mobility in our bodies and the environment. And mercury vapor is readily converted into the supercharged poison organic mercury by naturally-occurring bacteria found in bodies of water and in our own bodies.

Amalgam can kill people if handled improperly. The next story examines one such incident in Michigan in 1989.

Heating amalgam kills four, 1989

It was late August 1989. The place was Michigan. Four people -- two men and two women -- who lived in the same home lay dead.

Less than a month earlier, they were hospitalized after complaining of chest pain, diarrhea, nausea and shortness of breath. Their breathing became more labored and difficult. Four days into their hospital stay, it was learned that one of the men had been collecting mercury amalgam dental fillings. He had been heating them up in the basement so he could extract the small amount of silver from the fillings to sell. Substantial respiratory support, along with aggressive medical procedures to remove mercury from their bodies were initiated to no avail. All four died of mercury poisoning.

Their house was extensively cleaned in the hopes of removing the mercury. But the cleaning failed and the contaminated house was declared unfit for habitation. It had to be torn down.[276] We can only hope that the mercury laden rubble was disposed of as hazardous waste.

Those people died from breathing mercury vapor that came from heating the same type of fillings that are in 100 million Americans' teeth. Mercury amalgams are being placed into human beings at an alarming rate. It is estimated that 100 million new fillings containing mercury are placed in teeth each year in the U.S. alone.[277]

I am aware of no material except mercury amalgam that is used daily in our bodies by medicine or dentistry, that can contaminate whole buildings and kill people simply by being heated.

The material that killed these people is what you may be chewing on this moment. Chewing has been shown to dramatically increase the mercury vapor released from amalgams, due to the heat and friction generated from the pressure of chewing. One study found that more than 15 times the mercury vapor was released from amalgams after chewing as compared to non-chewing times.[278]

Other sources of mercury vapor are no less toxic. Mercury vapor from thermometer manufacturing has also taken its toll on American lives. One of the most moving stories I have ever read about work-related mercury contamination follows. It happened to be the cover story of *The New York Daily News Magazine* of March 15, 1987. Mercury vapor's ability to cause pain and suffering on many levels is revealed in this greed-induced tragedy.

Mercury madness in Brooklyn, 1987

Mercury poisoning and death haunted the workers of the Pymm thermometer factory in Brooklyn. One former employee recalled that he felt fine going to work in the morning, but within a few hours, he felt like the devil was inside him. He fought with his wife and tried to cut his father with a knife. Twice he tried to commit suicide. His nightmares were filled with blood. Even though he didn't work at the plant any more, he still shook, was forgetful, had a low appetite, lost weight, was going bald and had bleeding gums. He was diagnosed as suffering from excess mercury exposure. And he may have been one of the lucky ones. He was still alive.

Another worker was said to have suffered permanent brain damage. A pregnant employee who was advised by a doctor that her baby was at risk from the mercury decided to have an abortion. A 22-year-old man who only worked there one-and-a-half years had terrible headaches, stomach pain, earaches and lost 50 pounds. A 43-year-old woman fainted a lot and battled dizziness, memory lapses and mood swings. Another female worker began to lose her hearing. The story gets worse.

Three employees died. Tremors and weight loss preceded one woman's death from kidney failure, a documented result of mercury poisoning. A second woman, who had told co-workers about her headaches and vomiting in the bathroom, was found on the floor, foaming at the mouth during lunch hour. She was taken to the hospital, lapsed into a coma and died. No information was given on the third death.

Working conditions were described as extremely dangerous and violated OSHA regulations for nearly four years. OSHA simply slapped owners' hands through small fines and deadline extensions the whole time.

Many employees were afraid and reluctant to cooperate with investigators. And, interestingly, medical authorities said mercury exposure could have deepened the workers' reluctance to come forward because shyness, anxiety and timidity are symptoms of mercury poisoning.

The employees had no union, paid holidays or medical benefits. Many could not speak English and were not qualified for more skilled work. And, as incredible as it may seem, some workers were sent there by a mandatory federal workfare program. So they were afraid to lose what little job security they had by testifying against their employer.

The employees did agree, however, on one thing: greed caused the tragedy at the thermometer factory. Complying with the safety regulations would have cost money, cutting into the bottom line.

New York State Attorney General Robert Abrams and Brooklyn District Attorney Elizabeth Holtzman got criminal indictments against two of the plant's owners and the foreman. This was historic in that it was the first indictment to treat the alleged exposure to mercury as a violent crime committed by corporate executives.[279]

Health and safety must come before profit. How do any of us profit by the death of working people? Mercury is one of the most poisonous substances known to man. If it is treated as such, then sickness and death need not be a result of its use.

Government safety regulations work to our benefit in most cases. In Connecticut, the regulations did just that. Let's look at a case in that state where more than a thousand tons of soil were contaminated by mercury from dental amalgams.

Amalgams declared hazardous by EPA, 1983

In April 1983, children in Willington, Connecticut found a large area of mercury while playing with a metal detector. Their parents notified the Hazardous Materials Management Unit of the state Environmental Protection Agency (EPA). A second area of mercury contamination was discovered nearby. Both sites measured mercury concentrations from 17,000 parts per million (ppm) to as high as 29,000 ppm. (Tuna is removed from supermarket shelves when it has 1 part per million mercury.) The mercury in the soil came from dental amalgams. Scrap filling material (the part that was too much to fit into the tooth or was removed from the tooth) had been collected from dentists and dental supply companies for recycling. The contamination occurred during the recycling process. The EPA declared dental amalgam a hazardous substance and moved forward with plans to clean up the area.

According to a report in *Dentistry Today* on the incident,

> *"Jeremy Firestone, an assistant regional counsel at EPA in Boston, and the agency's chief lawyer in the case, stressed that 'the agency is not saying that amalgam is hazardous or toxic to anyone when it is in their mouths.'"*[280]

I always thought that what makes a substance hazardous or toxic was its chemical and toxicological properties rather than its location. So, Jeremy, amalgam is hazardous in my own backyard, but not in my mouth?

Dentists involved with selling the scrap amalgam were found to be partly liable for the contamination. Fifty-eight dentists across New England agreed out of court to pay partial damages. The cost to clean up 2.4 million pounds of soil was $700,000. The settlement from the dentists was almost $70,000. You and I, the taxpayers, picked up the other $630,000.[281,282]

Ott Dental Supply, one of the defendants, asked at what point do dental amalgams become hazardous and/or toxic substances. The answer was:

> *"Amalgam is always a hazardous substance within the meaning of Section 107 of CERCLA [Comprehensive Environmental Response Compensation and Liability Act]. Under the law, any material that contains a hazardous substance is itself a hazardous substance under Section 107 of CERCLA."*[283]

The lawyer for Ott was concerned that the EPA ruling declaring amalgams a hazardous substance would "open the floodgates of litigation. What makes it different in your mouth from when it's in your backyard? To me a hazardous substance is something you don't touch, eat or come into contact with."[284] That makes sense.

Giving mercury different labels does not change what it does. The mercury that goes in your mouth may be called a "filling" and the excess amalgam left on the dentist's tray after your filling is put in may be called a "hazardous substance" under the Superfund law. But they both leach mercury, one into the air and the other into your body.

In your medicine cabinet

You may be surprised to learn how many commonly found items in your medicine cabinet contain mercury, from mascara to hemorrhoid preparations. Calomel, mercury bichloride, ammoniated mercury, merbromin, ortho-hydroxyphenylmercuric chloride, phenylmercuric nitrate, and thimerosal are mercury compounds that have been used in over-the-counter products. Check the ingredients list for these names.

Even though the FDA placed all mercury ingredients for topical antiseptic use in "category II" early in 1982, many products still contain mercury. Category II labeling is for drug products not generally recognized as safe or effective for over-the-counter first aid use.[285]

When we were children, many of us were exposed to mercury compounds in Merthiolate and Mercurochrome. Let's find out more about these products.

Mercury-containing compounds: Merthiolate/Mercurochrome/Thimerosal

Do you recall scraping your knee from a bike accident and having your mom put Merthiolate or Mercurochrome on it? I always thought the orange-colored liquid hurt worse than the fall. It stung like crazy while my mom said, "Blow on it, that will make it feel better." Well, mom, it truly did not make it feel better.

What is Merthiolate or Mercurochrome anyway and why are they not around any more? Merthiolate is the trade name for thimerosal, an organic mercury compound. Mercurochrome is the trade name for merbromin, also an organic mercury compound.

In 1983, high blood mercury levels in several people and a death was reported from putting Merthiolate into ears. Shortly thereafter, the FDA banned the manufacture of Merthiolate due to safety concerns and a lack of evidence of effectiveness. However, on December 2, 1992, I called a local pharmacy and the pharmacist said that up until September, 1992, she was still able to order it. I find it hard to believe that the manufacturers had nine years of stock laying around in warehouses when the ban went into effect.

Mom thought she was helping to clean your knee when she was really using something now considered unsafe and ineffective.

We also once thought that the carcinogenic pesticide DDT was safe. The safety of DDT was not brought into question until Rachel Carson's bestseller <u>Silent Spring</u> helped launch an investigation. DDT was found to be poisonous to humans and the environment and was banned. I believe an impartial investigation into the safety of amalgam will result in its ban as well.

Merthiolate in my eyes

I was putting Merthiolate in my eyes for years and didn't know it. This story started in fourth grade when I got my first pair of glasses. Four-eyes in fourth grade. I had no idea anyone could see farther than a foot away, let alone across the room. It was the first time I could see the teacher writing anything on the blackboard. I also realized that my classmates in second grade did see me toss those blocks across the room. It was a humbling time for me. All those things I thought I had gotten away with were seen clearly by almost everyone else.

I had a heavy prescription for nearsightedness, so my glasses made dents in my nose. I remember being called four-eyes and having my glasses stomped by a bully in seventh grade. I now realize he had problems of his own, demonstrated by his need to destroy my glasses. He is probably undergoing therapy today. (His name was Steve. Steve, if you're reading this, relax. I forgive you.) Another thing I noticed about my glasses was that they seemed to have a sign on them, visible only to pretty girls, saying, "Don't date me."

Boy, was I glad to get my first pair of contact lenses in high school. Contacts erased the dents on my nose and assisted my quest to know the fairer sex. My contacts were great, except for one problem. Whenever I used the store-bought contact lens solutions, my eyes got very bloodshot, dry and sore. Back then, contact lens solutions (used for rinsing and storing) contained thimerosal, an organic mercury compound used as a preservative. Merthiolate is the trade name for thimerosal. I was putting Merthiolate in my eyes. It's no wonder they hurt. So I made my own saline with salt and distilled water. That worked just fine for me.

I was not alone in experiencing eye problems with thimerosal. It seems eye irritations ranging from mild to severe were happening to a lot of people using saline containing mercury. As early as 1983, it was known that up to 50% of contact lens wearers in the United States were affected.[286] Some users of thimerosal developed sensitivity years after non-symptomatic use.[287]

The saline manufacturers started making solutions for "sensitive eyes." It would have been more correct to label the new solutions "for eyes sensitive to mercury preservatives," but it sounds better to have a solution for sensitive eyes because that conveys a sense of concern, a special sensitivity that makes the manufacturer look good. I feel safe in saying most everyone's eyes are sensitive. An eyelash in the eye feels like a log.

The dilution factor of thimerosal in most solutions was 1:10,000 (one hundred parts per million). At this concentration, numerous effects were seen in eyes. This same dilution of thimerosal is used in many children's vaccines today. (see Vaccines, page 145)

Another place you may not expect mercury to be hidden is in batteries that power your children's toys.

Mercury in kids' toys; first mercury-free batteries from Eveready

If you have children, you probably have batteries in toys. If you have batteries in toys, you may have mercury in the batteries. The Eveready Battery Company received one of *Popular Science's* prestigious "100 Greatest Achievement Awards in Science" for the mercury-free battery and related discoveries. Until June 1991, all alkaline and carbon/zinc batteries had mercury in them. When they were disposed of, they either went into landfills or were incinerated. Neither method was satisfactory to Eveready. Batteries in the landfill rupture, spilling mercury into the environment. Incinerated batteries pollute the air with mercury vapor. Eveready took years of research and spent millions of dollars to develop its mercury-free battery.[288] Eveready, I salute your foresight and concern for the health of the consumer and the planet. Other companies have joined Eveready in making mercury-free batteries. You can help the environment by buying mercury-free batteries.

Mercury is a good electrical conductor. That is why it is in batteries, fluorescent bulbs and electrical switches. Did you know mercury switches were used in those sneakers that light up?

Foot in mouth

Athletic shoes containing lights in their soles were banned by the Minnesota Pollution Control Agency. Why would a pollution control agency ban athletic shoes? Because the motion switches inside the shoes were made with mercury. Agency officials banned the shoes out of concern over health hazards to animals from the used, thrown-out shoes. Once the shoes are in the landfills, mercury can leach into the soil and water. Each pair of the shoes contains about one gram of mercury for the switches.[289] Ironically, a large dental amalgam filling can contain as much as three grams of mercury.

I say recycle the shoes. Save them for your next dental filling! Your dentist can just cut the shoe open and mix the mercury with the silver alloy powder, making the traditional amalgam. Since you are saving the dentist material costs, you should request a discount. If the dentist is truly astute, he or she will realize your dedication to recycling and to protecting wildlife. Taking that a step further, the dentist may be clever enough to advertise the uniqueness of the practice:

"Dedicated to recycling and to protecting our wildlife, Dr. Oldshoe is in step with the belief that one must always put one's best foot forward. At our office, putting your foot in your mouth saves money. We like to say our fillings have sole."

Okay, so I'm getting sarcastic. Well, it just seems so blatantly obvious that if there is a problem with one gram of mercury in the discarded shoes, then there is a problem with three grams of mercury in a filling. Are we concerned with wildlife eating our shoe's mercury and not about humans ingesting fillings' mercury? I think a review of priorities is in order.

Let's now look at dental schools and dental offices. Are they polluted with mercury? Does the pollution in dental offices stay there or is it spread into our environment?

Your dentist's office; is it safe?
Mercury allergies caused by dental amalgam

In 1972-73, dental students at the University of Texas Dental Branch at Houston were tested for the development of mercury hypersensitivity during their four years at school (hypersensitivity reactions can include skin rashes, kidney problems, fever, arthritis, muscular pain and enlarged spleen or enlarged lymph nodes).[290] The results clearly showed that more than a **five-fold increase of mercury hypersensitivity developed** as students went through dental school.

In my dental school, we used mercury amalgam very little during the first year. So these increases in hypersensitivity could be more accurately seen over three to three-and-a-half years. Practicing dentists are exposed to much more amalgam than students and dental careers can easily span 30 to 50 years.

The Texas Dental Branch study concluded that mercury allergy in dentistry is caused by amalgam:

They said that no other source of mercury came close to the allergenic potential of amalgam. "Amalgam is by far the most significant source [of mercury hypersensitivity]."[291]

This study is important for two reasons. First, mercury allergy was produced by exposure to fillings outside the mouths of the students. If mercury can cause allergy in three years of dental school outside the mouth, what does it do in people with it inside the mouth for 20 or more years? Secondly, assuming dental schools are typical of the dental office, mercury exposure happens to everyone who goes into the dental office, the dentist, staff and patients.

Permanent nerve damage from dental mercury in office

An article in the *Journal of the American Dental Association* in June 1977 says that many dentists and their staffs are not well informed about mercury exposure hazards, contamination problems and effective clean-up procedures.

The article reports on mercury blood tests that were done on 111 dentists and dental staff during the Maryland Dental Convention meeting in September 1974, at Ocean City, Maryland. More than 50% had above-normal mercury levels. Test results indicated that mercury levels continue to rise in the blood with the number of years of exposure with no peak level.

In the same article, handwriting abnormalities were used as a possible indication of mercury toxicity. Seven participants had suspicious tremors. The highest blood levels of mercury did not necessarily correspond to the worst tremors. That is, blood levels were not found to be an indication of damage. Permanent brain damage from high mercury blood levels early in the dentists' careers was suspected to have caused the tremors.[292]

How can we justify the use of a filling material that can cause this kind of permanent damage at the beginning of a professional's career? Would you feel comfortable knowing that your dentist, who performs precise, delicate surgery on your teeth, has tremors from brain damage? How do you feel, knowing this unsteadiness could simply be due to breathing the office air poisoned by mercury coming off the fillings that he or she may have packed in your tooth?

My lawyer once told me of a case involving an older dentist who had such bad handwriting, he could not decipher his own notes in the courtroom.

Mercury exposure lowers dental skills

Can a dentist's continual exposure to mercury affect his or her performance? Read this from a government report:

". . . A team of researchers at the University of Michigan recently tested 142 volunteers from four plants that use mercury in the manufacture of chlorine or electronic materials. The workers, who had an average of 5 years exposure to mercury, were asked to perform such precise motor tasks as finger and toe tapping, button pressing, pencil flipping and following a maze with a stylus [pointer]. The scientists also measured muscle tremor while the volunteers held weights slung over their wrists. The tests were then repeated with a control group that had not been exposed to mercury. Results showed that the exposed workers had more trouble performing small, fast, repetitive movements; had slower tapping rates; and had more frequent muscle tremors. These are all indications that the mercury - even at low levels - was affecting the motor control centers of the brain."[293]

Dental work is a series of small, fast, repetitive movements that require a high degree of muscle control for accuracy. How many dentists have had their performance adversely affected by breathing mercury vapor in the office? How many dentists have had to retire from the profession due to uncontrollable tremors? And how many of those shaky-handed dentists would ever know their problem was from mercury used in dental amalgam?

Mercury spills, mental problems

Also in the same government report:

"One state occupational safety and health official tells of a laboratory where employees over the years had a strange history of mental problems. When the building was finally demolished, no less than 7 pounds of mercury were found under the laboratory floor!

Admittedly this is an extreme example of mercury build-up, but contamination still occurs -- even in what may seem the most unlikely places. For instance, recent medical tests of more than 100 Maryland dentists showed that two-thirds had high levels of mercury in their blood -- apparently as a result of inhaling vapors from mercury accidentally spilled during preparation of fillings. The mercury lodged in carpets or floor tiles in the dentists' offices and was not removed through normal cleaning."[294]

Does your dentist use mercury amalgam? Is there carpet in the treatment rooms? If even one drop of mercury was spilled on the carpet, the only way to clean it up is to remove the carpet. What are the chances of a dentist spilling mercury or pieces of amalgam on the carpet in one year, five or ten years? How long has your dental office used mercury fillings? The longer it has used mercury, the higher the potential contamination. Remember, mercury vapor has no taste or smell. Mercury vapor is impossible for human senses to detect.

A mercury spill in a California dental office

In the February 1984 issue of the *California Dental Association Journal* there is a story written by a dentist that describes a mercury spill in his office. It all started at four-thirty on a Friday afternoon. Dr. Metlen was waiting for an 11 year-old girl to get numb while he thought she was reading a book. His dental assistant came in to tell him that the little girl had walked across the treatment room and opened up the cap on the mercury reservior and poured mercury all over herself, the chair and the wall-to-wall carpet.

He entered the treatment room and found mercury all over the girl's clothes and in the chair. At first, he did not think much mercury had fallen on the carpet. But then he realized that the mercury had hit the carpet and broken into tiny droplets that sunk down and dissapeared into it. He described how mercury was dripping from her when she moved. He wanted to contain the mercury spill to one room if possible. So he decided that her mother should come into the room and remove all the girl's clothing and shoes in a plastic garbage bag. The child was given a dental smock and some towels to wear. He then let the mother and child take the plastic bag with the contaminated clothes and shoes home. The dentist told her mother not to open the bag and that he would call her to let her know what to do with the bag on the following Monday after he had talked with the health department.

Dr. Metlen closed up the office, went home and thought about what he should do. He literally paced up and down for hours. He thought he might just have the carpet replaced, but he knew that was illegal. The carpet handlers would not know to wear protection and would not know to dispose of the carpet according to hazardous waste guidelines. Besides, the chair was covered with mercury and needed very specialized cleaning. Fortunately, he had the wisdom to not do these things.

He worried that the mercury vapor build up in the office over the weekend would be too great, so he decided to call the Poison Control Center. They were unable to directly help, but gave him the phone number of a corporation that could clean up the mess. When he spoke with them, he decided to ask them to come out the next morning at nine o'clock, thinking he would save money if they did not work at night. He was told to get a permit from the state to bury hazardous waste. Dr. Metlen asked how much it might cost. He was told two to three thousand dollars. He said he almost passed out.

The next morning, the cleanup crew arrived promptly at nine. Two trucks, a station wagon, specialized equipment and what he described as "900 pounds of people" were ready to go. A man with a mercury vapor detector went into the contaminated office first, followed by the dentist and two other employees of the cleanup company. Suddenly the man with the detector told them all to stop. The meter on the detector was pegged at its highest reading and they were not even inside the closed door where the mercury was spilled, they were all instructed to go back outside.

Back outside, two men donned protective suits that covered their entire bodies. They went in and tore up the carpet piece by piece and placed it into a yellow oil drum marked "Hazardous Waste." The chair was washed with a chemical solution several times to decontaminate it. Everything that the men had worn while decontaminating the room was also tossed into the yellow drum.

On Monday, he spoke to the health department and the carpet people. He advised the mother that the health department said to simply wash the girl's clothes. They said that if the parents had any furthur concern they would send someone out to measure the mercury left in the child's clothes. Dr. Metlen had new carpet placed back into the same room. [294a]

The health department should have followed the same rules that applied to the mercury cleanup. The girl's clothes and shoes were contaminated and should have been disposed of as hazardous waste with the proper hazardous waste permit.

Dental office mercury levels above government limit

Another study reported in the *Journal of the American Dental Association* found that 37% of the dental operatories (patient treatment rooms) studied in San Antonio, Texas, had at least one mercury vapor measurement that exceeded the governmental limit, called the threshold limit value (TLV), for mercury exposure. In one treatment room, all 84 measurements were equal to or exceeded the TLV.

"Participants and auxilliary personnel were not aware of the degree of their continued exposure to mercury vapor contamination. As far as could be determined, this is the general situation throughout the dental profession."[295]

The TLV was set because of concerns over mercury as an atmospheric pollutant. Before 1974 the TLV was 100ug [100 millionths of a gram] of mercury per cubic meter of air. In 1974 the TLV was lowered by 50% to 50 ug of mercury per cubic meter of air. Apparently, newer technology determined that the old standard did not provide an adequate level of protection. This immediately brings to my mind the question: what if we find out again, with even newer technology, that this new TLV is still too high? What do we say to the people who were exposed to the supposedly safe TLVs? Sorry, we were wrong, you really were not safe?

The San Antonio study concludes that a systematic program of mercury vapor monitoring should be done by all offices using mercury. Does your dentist have a mercury monitoring program in effect?

I don't know of a single dental office that does this. Yet the technology is available.[296]

Mercury vapor inhaled by all who enter office

Everyone who walked into any of the dental offices in this last study were exposed to poisonous mercury vapor. But the exposure can run even wider than that. Anyone in any room in the building that has a common air circulation with the polluted areas could be breathing mercury vapor. For example, let's say a mother takes her sick child to visit a doctor who happens to have an office in the same building as a dentist that uses mercury. If, as in many cases, the air circulation system is shared by the whole building, then the sick child may be breathing mercury vapor.

There is no way a person can detect through the senses if he or she is being exposed to mercury vapor. It has no color, taste or smell. And what about the pregnant woman seeing her Ob-Gyn for her monthly checkup in the same sick building? What about the senior citizen waiting for the rheumatologist -- or the severly depressed adolescent waiting for his counseling appointment?

The many ways mercury vapor is released in dental offices

An article in *Florida Environments* of July 1993, titled "Metal, Chemical Hazards Rampant in Dental Offices" (sent to me by a geologist patient) describes many ways mercury vapor can be released into office air. For example, mercury vapor escapes while mixing amalgam, while putting amalgam in the tooth, during removal of old amalgams and during amalgam polishing. Since roughly 75% of all dental restorations are mercury amalgams, chances are high these mercury-releasing procedures are happening a lot of the time in the typical dental office.

Pieces of uncovered amalgam release mercury for extremely long periods. Small pieces of amalgam in the carpet or elsewhere can pose a serious mercury vapor problem.[297] Amalgam scraps dropped in the carpet, behind a cabinet or in the crack of a drawer, emit mercury 24 hours a day for 40 or more years. Maybe the last patient in the chair had four or five new mercury amalgams placed. Maybe some new amalgam pieces are still in the room, dropped on the carpet, or in the seam of the headrest.

I took out the carpet in my office and, although I am mercury-free, the dentist before me was not. I replaced the carpet with seamless surgical-grade flooring that runs up the walls several inches to allow for easier cleaning. My staff and I all noticed how much cleaner the office feels. My patients love the new floor and benefit through our increased ability to sanitize the treatment rooms.

Normal office cleaning does not remove the mercury from the carpet or floor tiles. According to one study, two thirds of Maryland dentists and dental technicians had high mercury blood levels. The high readings were thought to be caused by inhaling mercury vapors from accidental spills during the preparation of amalgam.[298]

Mercury vapor is known to soak into plaster walls to a depth of 10 cm.[299] Ten centimeters is nearly four inches. There is no known way to remove mercury from plaster walls other than removing the plaster. This could lead to expensive renovations in some offices.

How long has mercury been used in your dentist's office? Has the office been a dental office for generations? Was your new doctor's office a dental office prior to becoming a medical office? Do you work in an office that used to be a dental office? How many known or unknown spills occurred during the years mercury had been used in the office? In a truly mercury-free office, mercury spills are impossible.

Mercury hazards rampant

According to one estimate, about 10% of the dental offices in the United States exceed the mercury Threshold Limit Value (TLV) as a result of poor mercury handling practices.[300] How many more are near the limit? And what about dental schools where mercury handling techniques are not as refined because the students are inexperienced?

Is your dentist in the ten percent that exceeds our government maximum TLV? Or does your dentist practice mercury-free dentistry? If your dentist uses mercury fillings, the office has mercury vapor in the air.

Mercury poisoning symptoms may be ignored

An article in the *New York State Dental Journal,* looked at studies that examined the problems associated with mercury exposure in the dental office. It says that chronic mercury poisoning is difficult to diagnose because symptoms develop gradually over time and that often, with the exception of tremors, the symptoms may be ignored or blamed on other causes. This is particularly true in cases of mercury erethism, a condition characterized by irritability, outbursts of temper, excitability, shyness, resentment of criticism, headache, fatigue, and indecision. Another condition called micromercurialism accounts for psychological disturbances found in persons exposed to the concentrations found in most of the dental offices surveyed. Micromercurialism symptoms include loss of memory, irritability, fatigue, loss of self esteem and depression.[301]

Bizarre behavior

Why are dentists often described as having odd personalities? The answer seems clear: chronic exposure to mercury in their place of business. So many dental assistants have told me of the bizarre behavior of some of the dentists with whom they have worked. One assistant described her boss as a very nice man, who would suddenly have outbursts of anger, often throwing dental instruments across the room when something went even a little bit wrong. She left him because of his increasingly unpredictable behavior. Slight variations on this story are common.

The first signs of chronic mercury poisoning are usually behavioral. Irritability, anxiety, sleep disturbances, headaches, fatigue, short-term memory loss, tension and depression are common indicators of mercury poisoning. Even the American Dental Association recognizes these and other symptoms for mercury exposure. In its 1984 recommendations on dental mercury hygiene the ADA included the following signs and symptoms of mercury exposure: depression, fatigue, increased irritability, moodiness, nervous excitability, insomnia, headaches, nausea, loss of appetite, red patches on the skin, diarrhea, lung infections, kidney problems, swollen glands, swollen tongue, mouth ulcers, loosening of teeth, difficulty in fine hand movements like handwriting [and dental procedures], and tremors progressing to convulsions.[302,303,304,305]

How much depression among dentists and their staff is a direct result of their daily exposure to mercury amalgam? In one study of mercury in the blood of mental patients, referred to earlier in this book, elevated levels were found in a number of cases, especially among those with depression and severe mental problems.[306]

If you care about your dentist and the dental staff, ask them to stop using mercury. I'm sure if enough patients express a concern, compliance will follow. You can help your dentist to stop exposing himself or herself to the serious risks of mercury vapor.

Mercury from dental offices does find its way into our environment. The next few pages explain how this happens.

The environment, inside and outside my office

I believe that health-centered dentistry includes more than a good dentist. It includes the bigger picture of how the dental office fits into

177

the environment and how the environment fits into the office. Here is what I do in my office (and I'm always open to further suggestions):

• My treatment rooms have seamless, medical-grade flooring extending up the walls four inches for easy clean-up.

• I recycle aluminum, plastic and newspaper from the office, even though it means taking those items home. A little effort from a lot of people makes a huge difference to our environmental future. My little recycling effort is part of the huge difference.

• The office is cleaned using natural, biodegradable cleaning products.

• Special ionizing filters are in the intakes of the air conditioning/heating system. Indoor air is invariably more polluted than outdoor air. Ionizing filters keep the indoor air quality high.

• During the day, additional ionizing filters run in each treatment room. That is because more dust is created in the treatment rooms during working hours. These additional filters keep the air quality high even during busy days. And in the middle of the office, a large ionizing filter runs 24 hours a day.

• At night, an ozone generating unit cleans the air. Ozone kills bacteria and viruses and burns pollutants out of the air.

• Distilled water is offered to patients for rinsing.

• My staff and I choose the color of our scrubs so as to convey an atmosphere of calmness, professionalism and trust. Our current colors are deep purple and royal blue.

• The plants in the office are not just attractive; they add oxygen to the air and filter out contaminating organic vapors.

• I choose post-consumer waste, chlorine-free recycled tissue products for office use.

• The office is outfitted with energy-saving and workplace-enhancing full spectrum fluorescent lighting.

• We asked our dental supply houses to not use plastic packing materials for shipping and instead to use newspapers or other recyclable paper materials. They agreed.

• The paint used on the walls was selected for its lack of volatile organic solvents.

• The glue used on our carpet was also selected for its lack of volatile organic solvents.

• And we use natural fiber upholstery where possible.

WATER SUPPLY CONTAMINATION BY DENTAL MERCURY

Mercury amalgam disposal is unmonitored

If you thought lead in your water was bad, try mercury. Remember, lead and mercury poisoning symptoms are identical. Mercury from dental amalgam finds its way into wastewater from dental offices, and some wastewater is being recycled.

Disposal of mercury amalgam from the dental office is currently unmonitored. And although many dentists are conscientious about recycling,

" . . . problems can arise when mercury fillings are disposed of down drains which eventually enter septic tank systems. This practice may pose a threat to adjacent groundwater quality. Also, poor disposal practices of used fillings and other mercury-containing wastes may lead to potential soil (and perhaps even groundwater) contamination."[307]

ADA fighting regulation of mercury waste

A prominent article in the February 21, 1994 issue of the *Journal of the American Dental Association* was typical of the ADA's response to regulation of its favorite filling material, amalgam. In it, the ADA admitted that studies done across the United States show that up to

15% of all mercury contamination found in water treatment facilities comes from dental offices. And they acknowledged that the EPA had already identified dental amalgam as an environmental threat. But their response was not concern for the safety of the environment or personal health, but rather concern about more regulations for dentists. The title of the article was "ANOTHER REGULATION? State, local officials scrutinizing amalgam waste in water supplies."

Until 1993, the ADA did not even address environmental dental mercury issues. Now, with the threat of regulations, they have seen a need to be involved. The newly formed Waste Management Task Force, co-headed by the Division of Legal Affairs, formalized the ADA's involvement. In the article, the following paragraph described the ADA's view on the task force's duties:

"The group is charged with monitoring environmental issues that could affect dentists and investigating the scientific basis of potential regulations on dental waste."[308]

Not a single word in the article even alluded to protecting environmental or personal health! The entire point of the task force seems to be to protect dentists from regulations. Mercury from dental offices is being dumped without any questions into our water treatment plants and septic tanks. The task force was created to slow down the regulative machinery by questioning the validity of each and every step in the regulatory process. The ADA goes so far as to say,

" '. . . Any regulation -- if one is warranted at all -- should be site specific.' What might be needed in one town . . . could be far different for what's called for in a city two or three hundred miles away."[309]

Let me ask what newly discovered law of toxicology says that a poison in one town is far different than the same poison in a city two to three hundred miles away?

" 'I'm worried about being forced to install some sort of expensive amalgam separator,' " said the president of the San Francisco Dental Society in the article.[310]   Again, not a word of concern for your health or the environment, only for her checkbook.

It is simple and inexpensive to trap amalgam particles from effluent [discharged fluids] in plastic containers for proper disposal so that very little mercury is expelled into wastewater. The environmental health costs we all pay far outweigh the small cost incurred by dentists in keeping our water and soil free of dental mercury.

The reason dentistry exists is to protect personal health. Personal health greatly depends on the health of our environment. What we do with our waste is vitally important; it affects us all. Dentists are generating mercury waste products, materials which are indeed environmental threats. The profession, then, must accept responsibility for their safe disposal.

Better yet, if mercury is not used, it will not pose a health threat. The dental profession can't spill hazardous waste if they don't have it to spill. Since safer, better replacements are readily available, why not use them?

In the same article, the executive director of the ADA, John S. Zapp said,

" 'We already have involvement with key legislative committee members and their staffs, and we will aggressively be delivering the ADA's message.' "[311]

Who will be aggressively delivering the environmental or personal health message? The answer is you, the consumer. You can tell your dentist you refuse to have mercury put in your body. And you can contact your legislator and express your views on dental mercury waste regulation. If you think regulation is a good idea, speak up. The ADA is certainly promoting its biased views.

Chapter 5

Dental offices closed due to mercury contamination in wastewater

Dental offices in Tucson, Arizona, were closed recently due to excessive mercury contamination in their wastewater. In Seattle, the upper limit of mercury allowed in dental wastewater was exceeded by 750 times.[312]

How prevalent is dental mercury pollution? Dentists in the United States are estimated to use between 100 and 165 tons of mercury per year.[313,314] No one knows for sure, but estimates of the dental mercury used each year in North America that may end up in the wastewater run as high as 40%.[315] This percentage means that 80,000 to 132,000 pounds of mercury may be contributed by American dentists to wastewater contamination each year. And wastewater treatment leaves mercury contamination untouched, flowing into our lakes, aquifers, streams and coastal waters.

Wastewater treatment leaves toxic material untouched

In my home state of Florida alone, two billion gallons of wastewater from treatment plants discharge into lakes and coastal waters each year. Wastewater treatment does not keep toxic products from polluting our environment. Florida had 4.5 million homes and thousands of businesses hooked into the water treatment facilities in 1992. There currently is no way to determine how much toxic material flows out of these sources into the treatment plants.

The majority of the pollution in wastewater comes from households and small business, not big business. People dump toxins into the wastewater either on purpose or unknowingly, and we all wind up paying for this recklessness or ignorance. We pay for the cleanup costs, if it can be cleaned up at all. We pay in terms of environmental degradation. And we pay in terms of human health.

182

Not only do smaller wastewater treatment plants lack equipment capable of removing toxic pollutants, but larger plants as well. In 1991, the U.S. General Accounting Office stated that, in general, wastewater treatment does not remove toxic substances.[316] Mercury is a toxic substance.

There are almost 10,000 licensed dentists in Florida and improper use and disposal methods of mercury amalgam could pose a serious threat to the environment. Not only can it drop into cracks and carpets, vaporizing for a very long time, as we have learned, but it can enter septic tank systems which may contaminate nearby soil and groundwater.[317] Dental offices that use amalgam and have septic tanks may expose nearby well water to mercury pollution. Septic tank drain fields can drain toxic material into the groundwater supply. Just because it goes down the drain, doesn't mean it disappears. As a matter of fact, it may come back to us sooner than you think.

What we flush, we will drink

The squeeze on water supplies is growing tighter by the day. Water sources in many parts of the country are at or near the maximum use levels. Especially hard hit are larger cities undergoing growth. The U.S. Geological Survey estimated in 1985 that Americans' daily usage of fresh water averaged 1,400 gallons per person, including water used to cool power plants as well as to steam vegetables. The U.S. population growth is expected to exceed 11% from 1990 to 2000. That would add 26 million people, consuming an additional 36.4 billion gallons of water each day. It is clear to see, we don't have much choice other than recycling wastewater into drinking water. [318]

The Environmental Protection Department in Orange County, Florida must know something about drinking water. It allows 7.5 times the amount of lead in drinking water than it does mercury. And it allows 25 times the amount of arsenic in drinking water than it does mercury. [318a] They know that mercury is 7.5 times more dangerous than lead and 25 times more dangerous than arsenic in our drinking water.

Some states began experimenting with wastewater recycling plans many years ago. The Northern Virginia Upper Occoquan Sewerage Authority has recycled wastewater since June 1978. The process is called "potable reuse," probably because the term "recycled wastewater" did not have the same sound in the consumers' ear. Denver, Colorado, built a million-gallon-a-day potable reuse demonstration plant which consistently produced water quality equal to or better than the existing water supply. San Diego also has a water reuse research project. It demonstrated that the contamination risk from the recycled water system, called Aqua II, is equal to or less than that from the existing water supply. Tampa and San Diego have moved toward wastewater recycling. [319]

The main way our bodies get rid of mercury is through the feces; up to 20 times the rate released in urine. One recent study demonstrated a huge difference between people with and without amalgams. Those with amalgams had up tp 100 times greater fecal mercury concentrations than those without amalgams.

The vast majority of treatment plants do not remove mercury from wastewater. So, mercury from dental amalgams pollutes the sludge (sometimes sold as fertilizer) and the recycled water. Products such as brake fluid, industrial cleaners, paint solvents and dental mercury in the wastewater will make it much harder for recycling plants to discharge pure drinking water. It is common sense to not let these nasties get into the water in the first place. If dentists don't use mercury, and there is no need to, the contribution dental mercury now makes to the pollution problem will disappear.

Dental procedures are driven by you, the dental consumer. You have the power to change the use of mercury in fillings. Tell your dentist, "I don't want mercury fillings in my teeth or my family's teeth." Demand the better filling materials - ask for composite resins.

In terms of chemical and electrical biocompatability, strength, wear, and color matching, nothing is better than composite resins. Consumers have the clout to change dentistry. By refusing to allow mercury in your body, you can make amalgam history and protect our water at the same time.

"If we pass the Everglades test, we get to keep the planet."

Joe Podgor, founder of Friends of the Everglades, spoke these words, meaning that if we learn the lessons presented to us by the Everglades, we can use them to solve other environmental problems. The Everglades National Park in south Florida is our country's second largest and most endangered park. The United Nations ranks its importance with the Egyptian pyramids and Africa's Serengeti. But its future is in jeopardy. And the greatest threat to its survival is pollution from mercury.[319a]

There are other threats to the Everglades besides mercury, although they are not as severe. Trees not commonly found in the Everglades, called exotics, have been introduced into the delicate habitat and are creating forests where there was only grass. Thirty square miles of grass have been replaced by Brazilian pepper trees. At the edges of the river of grass, real estate developers are changing the landscape. Shell Oil is trying to see how much money the poor Miccosukee Indians living in the Everglades will accept to allow oil drilling on their land. What truly amazes me is that our U.S. Postal Service has already parceled out zip codes for the Everglades. What is today a precious national park may be just another development tomorrow.[320]

Hurricane Andrew, the nation's most costly storm, stomped a 30-mile-wide swath through the Everglades. It blew down nearly all the tropical hardwood hammocks in its path and closed the park for a while.

Still, the largest threat to the Everglades is mercury pollution.[321]

Some of this comes from dental mercury amalgam burned in incinerators and crematoria. More than 50% of Florida's mercury pollution comes from incinerators. Most mercury from incinerators vaporizes into the air, but some is buried in landfills as ash.

Just two generations ago, there were ten times the number of birds in the Everglades. Today, once-abundant wildlife is having trouble surviving. Elevated mercury levels have been found in alligators, panthers, wood storks, bald eagles, brown pelicans, woodcocks, red-tailed hawks, ospreys, loons and herons.[322]

How mercury pollutes the Everglades

As more mercury gets into the Everglades from polluted rain or landfill runoff, it gets into the bottom of the food chain. Then, each time larger animals feed on the smaller creatures, they take in more mercury. The animals at the top of the food chain, such as the endangered Florida panther, eat many animals that eat other smaller animals. As a result, they are most at risk of high mercury levels. One panther died with mercury levels higher than the victims of the mercury-poisoning disaster in Minamata Bay, Japan (see "Minamata Disease," page 192). Warning signs posted in the Everglades tell fishermen not to eat bass caught there. Bass are near the top of the food chain and have been found with high mercury levels.

More than two million acres in the Everglades are affected by mercury contamination.[323] How much is contaminated with mercury from dental amalgam? How much more are we going to allow to be contaminated from dental fillings? The dangers of mercury used in dentistry affect our health, and the health of one of the world's most important bodies of water.

300% increase in mercury levels

The Orlando Sentinel newspaper conducted a year-long investigation into the state's groundwater contamination and found that mercury levels in the Everglades rose 300% in the last three to five years prior to 1992. The tested areas were far from any industrial source and the pollution was determined to be airborne.[324] Most of Florida's mercury pollution comes from incinerators which may burn batteries, switches, fluorescent bulbs, thermometers and dental mercury amalgam.

Floridians were warned by state agency officials to limit their consumption of fish caught in mercury-contaminated areas.[325] South Florida has the worst mercury pollution in the United States. Two children of south Florida resident Steve McClain tested above the safety level for mercury. McClain said:

" 'For my children to have this high a concentration a year after eating this fish, I wonder about the people who take fish home in buckets and eat it every day.' "[326]

Mercury levels in contaminated fish in the Everglades have been measured to be 50% higher than the FDA' s unsafe level.[327]

Widespread mercury pollution

Mercury contamination in America's lakes and rivers is widespread. A study by Clean Water Action and Clean Water Fund found that 26 states have issued health advisories for mercury-tainted fish. The worst contaminations were in Florida, Michigan, Minnesota, Wisconsin and New England.[328]

On Dec. 15, 1992, the Florida Department of Health and Rehabilitative Services (HRS), the Game and Fresh Water Fish Commission, and the Department of Environmental Regulation issued health advisories for 68 Florida waterways because of hazardous mercury levels. Twenty-two waterways in one year alone had been added to the list.[329] I called Florida's HRS Public Information and asked how many waterways were under a health advisory because of mercury contamination. One toxicologist said it would be much easier to tell me the waterways unaffected by the mercury poisoning than the ones that were.

Later that day, I spoke with Dr. Roberta Hammond, biological administrator, Environmental Epidemiology for the state of Florida, and asked if she would help me get answers to the following questions:

• How many cases of mercury poisoning from eating fish were reported in Florida during 1991, 1992 and 1993?

• How many cases of mercury poisoning due to fish consumption were reported in the United States during 1991, 1992 and 1993?

Shortly thereafter, I received a call from Dr. Tom Atkinson, mercury coordinator for the Florida Department of Environmental Protection. He said he was not aware of a single **reported** case of Acrodynia (mercury poisoning) from fish consumption in 1991, 1992, or 1993 in the North American continent.

Almost every single freshwater lake tested in the U.S. in 1991 was under a mercury advisory.[330] And all the literature I have read in 1994 suggests that the mercury pollution problem is getting worse rather than better. So how is it that not one person has been reported as getting sick from eating tainted fish for these three years? Common sense tells me that people must be getting sick from mercury poisoned fish, given the number of Americans that eat fish they catch. It seems obvious then, that these people are undiagnosed and misdiagnosed. I'm certain this is directly related to the difficulty in distinguishing mercury toxicity symptoms from those of other illnesses.

The highest levels of mercury are found in commonly caught gamefish such as bass, walleye, trout, pike, carp and catfish. These fish are often eaten. The Florida panthers that died from suspected mercury poisoning ate fish contaminated with high levels of mercury. I would not doubt that there are panthers in the Everglades right now that are ill because of mercury poisoning.

Who wants to be the doctor that diagnoses mercury poisoning from Florida bass just before the fishing or tourist season? What would the media do with that information? Florida's main business is tourism.

If you went to your doctor's office complaining of anxiety, moodiness and fits of anger, do you think the doctor would ask about your fish-eating habits? "Say, I hear you are irritable lately. Have you been eating fish caught down in the Everglades?" Or let's suppose you had hearing or vision disturbances along with memory loss or tingling in your feet. Would your physician suspect mercury poisoning? How many doctors do you suppose are aware of the need for hair analysis to determine organic mercury exposure? Mercury exposure symptoms vary so widely, and mock those of so many more common ailments, it is difficult to imagine mercury poisoning even being considered as a first diagnosis in most cases. It took medical experts 3 years to prove that mercury was the source of poisoning in Minamata Bay, Japan.[330a]

An HRS brochure states that mercury contamination from manmade sources (such as industrial pollution and coal and trash burning) release much more mercury into the environment than natural sources (oceans and natural ore deposits of red mercuric sulfide, called cinnabar). And mercury contamination in soil or air eventually ends up in water. [331]

What an ominous statement. **Any mercury pollution in soil or air, created by any source, eventually ends up in our water.** It seems the wisest thing to do would be find alternatives to mercury whenever possible. Roughly 100 tons of mercury each year are used by American dentists. Yet, dentistry has already found superior alternatives to mercury fillings -- composite resin fillings. We can protect ourselves and our precious environment at the same time using these composite fillings instead of mercury.

189

Dental mercury use contributes to global atmospheric pollution

Estimates on mercury released into the atmosphere each year, natural and manmade, range from 13 to as high as 81 million pounds. Guesses of man's contribution range from 10% to 80%. Regardless of what is true in terms of the numbers, natural sources of mercury are thought to remain relatively constant. Yet, global mercury pollution continues to rise. It is thought that the reason must be from the rise in manmade mercury pollution.

Fortunately, in the United States, between 1980 and 1990, mercury in batteries has decreased 90%, mercury in paint has been outlawed and even the total number of mercury fillings has decreased somewhat. Unfortunately, world-wide mercury pollution continues to increase, even though its use in the U.S. has decreased. A ban on mercury fillings would have a positive impact on global pollution.

World's largest case of dental mercury pollution unfolding today

The largest case of dental mercury pollution is happening in the Amazon jungles. How much devastation will be left in its wake is unknown.

Brazil using dental mercury for gold mining

Mercury is being used by miners in the Amazon basin to extract gold from river banks. Mercury is attracted to gold, and the miners use it to draw out gold from the river bank mud slurry. They then heat the gold-mercury combination to vaporize off the mercury, leaving the gold. Some mercury goes into the atmosphere, some washes into the river beds.[332]

A pound of mercury for every pound of gold

Brazilian biologist Sandra Hacon has estimated that for every pound of gold recovered there has been at least one pound of mercury released into the environment. Estimates of mercury dumped from 1982 to 1992 range between two and three million pounds. The extent of wildlife and human poisoning in the Amazon could well be the worst in history. Tens of thousands of people are disabled or dying from mercury exposure in the mining area.[333,334]

Dr. Xoltan Annau, a well-respected mercury toxicologist from Johns Hopkins University, went to review the gold mining operations at the request of the Brazilian government. He discovered that most of the miners were lawless, sometimes shooting and killing anyone they pleased.[335] This may be a link between mercury poisoning and violence that cries out to be studied. Science knows mercury poisoning can cause severe personality disturbances such as fits of anger and sudden mood swings. So mercury-induced violence, over and above the greed-induced violence, seems likely.

Annau found mercury literally covering the banks and beds of the river being mined. No attempt at cleaning it up was being made. The majority of the miners sold the gold to get cash to trade in cocaine. And the level of violence and ruthlessness was such that Annau's guides would not allow him to remain in mining areas beyond 4 p.m. The World Health Organization declined an invitation to send a group into the mining areas because of the danger.[336]

This terrible example of pollution-for-greed harms us all, not just the miners and the local inhabitants. Follow this pollution path. It leads back to the dental profession's use of mercury. Mercury released into the environment by man spreads in water, air and soil. Through air and water movement, mercury can be carried far away from the pollution source. The ocean will eventually get a lion's share of this mercury. What will we do if the oceans die from our mercury abuse? At what point is it too late? When will action be taken to stop such insanity?

Importing mercury for mining purposes was banned by Brazil. Yet, Brazilian importers are currently buying 680,000 pounds each year supposedly for dental purposes.[337] This amount of mercury is roughly 3.4 times the mercury used for dental purposes in the United States each year. Indisputably, the mercury is being purchased by the importers for use other than dental fillings. The miners are using dentistry to skirt the law.

I hope the ADA will take a stand against this massive abuse of dental mercury in the Amazon. When the pollution being created today in the Amazon enters the atmosphere and the oceans, it will affect us all. This devastation is due to the easy availability of dental mercury and human greed.

If we clean up the Amazon, do we get to keep the planet?

There have been other very serious environmental mercury disasters during this century. The most infamous crisis occurred in Minamata Bay, Japan.

Minamata Disease, 1956

I remember, when I was young, hearing the news about numerous people having birth defects, brain damage and premature deaths in Minamata Bay, Japan. It is now known as Minamata Disease it is not a disease, it is mercury poisoning.

From 1932 to 1968, the Chisso factory dumped an estimated 200-600 tons of mercury compounds into Minamata Bay and a tributary river.[338] People living on the bay ate fish and shellfish from the contaminated water. Babies were born with cerebral palsy, convulsions, slow reflexes, retarded body growth, speech disorders, mental retardation, limb deformities, hyperactivity, crossed eyes and spastic muscle twitching. Small heads were seen in 60% of the babies and the death rate was 7%. Most of the pregnant women exposed to the organic mercury showed no signs of poisoning.[339,340] Birds dropped into the ocean while flying; pigs, cats and dogs went mad and died. Local people had coined the term "dancing cats" to describe the horrible way in which cats died of mercury poisoning. The cats would act as if they were intoxicated, salivating and staggering about. Without warning, convulsions would strike them and they would spin erratically in bizarre, contorted circles, falling down dead. By 1957-1958 there were no cats left in four areas around Minamata.[340a] **It took 24 years of pollution before the cause of the tragedy was discovered. And it took 12 more years for the mercury dumping to be stopped.** Even though the dumping had halted in 1968, the pollution took its toll. In 1976, 126 people from the Minamata Bay area died from mercury poisoning and over 800 had severe brain damage. By 1982, the number of people affected by the pollution rose to 1,773; nearly 500 of them died.[341] And the pollution created decades ago is still affecting people today.

The medical professionals took a long time to discover the source of the poisonings because the symptoms were so numerous and different from each other.

The people in Minamata died at a rate of 38%. Every other living creature that ate the fish had similar symptoms, including cats, dogs, birds, pigs and rats.[342]

More global mercury poisonings Japan, 1964

Unfortunately, Japan learned a second lesson of mercury poisoning in 1964. In Niigata, Japan, over 120 citizens were poisoned from the identical causes discovered in Minamata. Nineteen babies were born with brain damage, but their mothers showed no signs of poisoning. There was the sad case of a 14-year-old boy who ate a great deal of tainted fish and shellfish during 10 days in 1953. Seven years later, in 1960, he still could not attend school because he could not remember the alphabet. I wonder how he continues to suffer because of greed-induced mercury poisoning.

Chapter 5

Iraq, 1956, 1960 and 1972

Iraq experienced large-scale mercury poisonings in 1956, 1960 and 1972. The first involved more than 100 people who ate seeds treated with a fungicide containing an organic mercury compound. Fourteen died. The victims who lived experienced the same central nervous system disorders mentioned in Minamata disease as well as weight loss, deep pain in their muscles (especially in their hands, feet and genitals) and excessive thirst and urination. Electrocardiogram changes were also found in some cases as was degeneration of the optic (eye) nerve.

Four years later, in 1960, several hundred more Iraqis were reported poisoned from the same source. More than 22 died.[343]

Twelve years later, in 1972, 6,530 Iraqis were admitted to hospitals and 459 died after eating bread made from grain treated with a mercury fungicide. Unfortunately, the mercury poisoning lessons of 1956 and 1960 had not been learned.[344]

Pakistan, 1961

During 1961, in West Pakistan, flour and wheat seeds treated with a mercury fungicide poisoned more than 100 people. Four died, and unreported deaths were suspected. Some of those affected became permanently blind.

Guatemala, 1963, 1964, 1965

Guatemala also has had the misfortune of three successive mercury poisonings. In the wheat planting seasons of 1963, 1964, and 1965, what seemed to be a viral inflammation of the brain was reported. The symptoms included arm and leg paralysis, deafness, blindness, loss of consciousness and death. All tests for encephalitis turned out negative. Victims died at a rate of 44%. Finally it was found that the affected people were eating seeds treated with a mercury-containing fungicide.[345]

Tragedy strikes an American family of nine, 1969

Tragedy struck a family of nine in December 1969, in a small New Mexico town. Three of the children were hospitalized. All had vision disturbances, erratic behavior, walking difficulties and lethargy which led to coma. Preliminary diagnoses included multiple sclerosis; viral encephalitis; arsenic, lead, cadmium or mercury poisoning; and overdosage of tranquilizers or sedatives. The symptoms could have fit any of these causes. Then health experts discovered that the family, with the exception of the two youngest children, had eaten pork that had been fed seed treated with a mercury-containing fungicide. Three months later, the mother gave birth to a son who went into convulsions a few hours into his life. Just as in Minamata, the mother showed no signs of mercury poisoning. Unfortunately, the three hospitalized children remained severely and permanently disabled.[346]

Sweden bans mercury fungicide use on seeds, 1966

Sweden, after studying the mercury content of various foods, decided in 1966 to ban seed fungicides containing mercury. No decrease in productivity was noticed, but a large decrease of Swedish wildlife mercury contamination was observed.[347] Isn't it interesting that Sweden championed the lead in banning mercury from seeds just as it has championed the lead in banning mercury in dental fillings (see page 206)?

U.S. bans mercury in pesticides and paint, but not in fillings or vaccines

The U.S. banned mercury from most pesticides in 1976.

195

EPA bans mercury in interior latex paint, 1990

On August 20, 1990, the Environmental Protection Agency (EPA) ordered that mercury be removed from interior latex paint because an unacceptable level of mercury vapor was being released. In the previous year, a four-year-old boy developed mercury poisoning by breathing paint fumes in his home. His symptoms were near-fatal and included a drastic personality change, fever, rapid heart beat, sweating, severe leg cramps, and nerve dysfunctions resulting in him barely being able to move his arms and legs. He was hospitalized for months.

Prior to 1990, mercury was added to paint as a preservative to prolong the shelf life and prevent mildew. Mercury was not added for the consumer, it was added for big business profits. Though mercury was banned from paint manufacturing after August 20, 1990, paint manufactured before that date containing the same poisonous levels of mercury being outlawed -- could still be sold. Why was the paint not recalled? Because personal health took a back seat to the business interests of the paint industry?

A parallel between paint and fillings

There is an eerie parallel between the way the mercury-in-paint issue was handled and the way the mercury-in-fillings issue is being handled.

Let's look back to 1976. In that year, the EPA decided to let the paint industry continue to use mercury in latex paints. The EPA said that not enough was known about the effects of mercury, and that manufacturers had no effective alternatives that cost the same as mercury. But neither of these excuses was true. In the very same year the EPA banned mercury from most pesticide uses because of its toxicity. So enough was known about mercury to remove it from pesticides, but not enough was known to remove it from paint?

And what about effective alternatives? In April 1990, the *New York Times* said several major national paint producers had not used mercury in paint for years, and *The Orlando Sentinel* reported that a local Sears paint store had not carried mercury in their paint since 1975. My thoughts are that the paint industry must have had a very effective lobby with our politicians between 1976 and 1990. Somehow, the ban of mercury in paint was effectively delayed for 14 years.

There is a parallel in the dental industry. For years now there have been stronger, safer and more attractive alternatives to amalgam: composite resin fillings. Many composites have proven to be better filling materials than amalgam.[348] Composites have been used by thousands of dentists for more than 20 years. And each year surveys indicate dentists are using more composites. The number of dental amalgams placed in the U.S. has decreased from almost 160 million in 1979 to about 100 million in 1990.[349] Part of the reason is found in the broader use of composite resin fillings.

However, the ADA still insists there are no viable alternatives to amalgam. The ADA has a very effective lobby, so nothing of substance is being done about dental mercury at the federal level. How much longer will the ADA delay the ban of mercury fillings? It was able to reverse the ban on dental mercury imposed 160 years ago and is still going strong: what a lobby!

During the 14-year delay on mercury in paint, how many adults and children were made ill by that mercury? Do we have to wait until a child nearly dies to take action against a known poison? What was the real cost of using mercury in paint in terms of human health? How many people must get sick before a poison is removed from the market? Does it depend on the size and clout of the industry using the offending material? We must look at the entire picture of using a poison, not just the industry's bottom line. By the way, in 1990, paint manufacturing was a profitable and powerful $12 billion-dollar-a-year industry.[350]

The arguments for continuing to use mercury in dentistry are exactly the same as those used by the EPA and the paint industry in 1976. The EPA, ADA and dental manufacturers say that not enough is known about mercury's effects and no effective alternatives are available that cost the same as mercury. Neither one of these excuses are true. If mercury is too toxic to be used in paint and pesticides, how can it be considered completely safe in the human mouth as amalgam fillings? More than enough is known about the health perils of mercury exposure and the release of mercury from amalgam to uphold a ban.

The national average cost of a one surface amalgam filling is $51. The national average cost of a surface composite filling varies from $63 to $70 depending on whether it is on front or back teeth. [350a] However, because composites take longer to put in and the material costs to the dentist are greater than they are for amalgam, the net profit for a composite is less. I believe the real issue for the ADA is the lower profit to its member dentists, not the cost to the patient. Would you pay a little more for a superior, safe filling that was invisible?

What is the real cost of using mercury in dentistry in terms of human health? How many people must relate their stories of improved health on removing dental mercury before the EPA moves to protect personal health? How many other sites of contamination due to dental mercury waste must be discovered before the EPA takes action to protect our environment? Why is the ADA lobbying against regulations for mercury in dentistry? We must bring soil, air and water pollution issues and personal health issues up to the front of the mercury debate. Let's not get lost in the profit motives of the dental profession. By the way, according to Chris Martin of the ADA communications department, dentistry, in 1993, was a profitable and powerful $37.1 billion-dollar-a-year industry.

Protecting profit or protecting health?

The commonly accepted understanding is that the EPA is supposed to have evidence of safety before a product is allowed on the market rather than proof of its damage after it is already on the market. But I understand that many products were "grandfathered in" before the EPA was given the power to approve products. Amalgam was one of those products. I believe the EPA exists for the health and welfare of Americans, not for the bottom line of large industries such as paint manufacturing or dentistry. Amalgam is one product that I am sure would not pass EPA guidelines if it were introduced today.

P.S. Mercury in exterior latex paint

The amazingly contradictory path of the EPA on mercury use in paint forged on. Though mercury had been banned from interior latex paint by the EPA, the EPA said that the data were not conclusive enough to determine if mercury in exterior latex paint was a health risk, so mercury was allowed to be used in exterior latex paint.

As follow-up, the EPA warned consumers against using mercury-containing exterior latex paints indoors, and the paint industry was required to look into the problem. Was it the paint industry's job to police itself? How effective was that? Was the fox placed in charge of the henhouse? The EPA said it would take steps when they became necessary.[351,352,353] Apparently, steps did become necessary: on May 22, 1991, the EPA finally decided it would be prudent to also ban mercury in exterior latex paint. How many children, pets and loved ones became ill while the EPA waited to make its decision?

It is deplorable to note that the FDA still allows mercury to be used in dental fillings and added to many vaccines (see "Children's Vaccines Contain Mercury!," page 146). Mercury is added to prolong the shelf life of vaccines, so pharmaceutical companies could be more assured of selling the vaccine before it goes bad. Preservatives add to the quantity of shelf life, not the quality of the product.

Mercury was used in paint as a mold and mildew inhibitor and in pesticides because of its ability to kill insects. It was removed from both because of its human health costs. But it is still being used in amalgam fillings and vaccines. And vaccines and amalgams are put into the body intentionally. I don't want a mold or mildew inhibitor or an insecticide in my mouth or my bloodstream.

The good news used to be that mercury from your paint only lingered in the air for months. The bad news is that mercury from amalgam fillings may linger in your body forever.

Mercury exposure from amalgams greater than that from paint

The New England Journal of Medicine, on March 21, 1991, published a letter from Drs. Murray Vimy and Fritz Lorsheider from the University of Calgary, Alberta, Canada, explaining that the level of mercury exposure from dental amalgams is greater than that from latex paint in an enclosed room.

That means something is very wrong with dental amalgams.

Because mercury from dental fillings finds its way into the atmosphere, we all end up sharing this pollution when we breathe. How does mercury from fillings get into the air? That is one of amalgam's burning issues.

Burning issues: pollution from the living

There are no EPA mercury emission limits for solid waste incinerators. The incinerator down the street from your house or your child's school can belch out as much mercury from its trash as it wants because no one is keeping track.

Our government does set limits on the amount of mercury considered safe in solid waste. But it's impossible to tell how much mercury is in each trash truck driving down your street. When it takes only one battery in 12,000 pounds of garbage to put the entire six tons of trash over the mercury limit for solid waste, it is not hard to imagine nearly every garbage truck exceeding the limit. Just a few batteries from one house could do it. Or maybe a few old amalgam scraps from the neighborhood dentist. An average mercury filling contains the same quantity of mercury as a hearing aid battery. Dental mercury amalgam can end up in the garbage truck purposefully or inadvertently.[354]

The problem with mercury in the trash is two-fold. First, much of solid waste is incinerated and mercury winds up in the atmosphere, coming back to the ground as contaminated rain. Second, solid waste containing mercury in a landfill leaches the poison into the soil, where it eventually ends up in water, polluting fish, other wildlife and, eventually, humankind.

How does dental mercury find its way into the trash? It is difficult for dentists to find reprocessing companies that take amalgam scraps. Scrap amalgam is not worth much and some refiners refuse to take it. Pieces of amalgam left over from placing new fillings can't be used again. As a result, they may be tossed into the trash because they are so inexpensive and it's the easiest thing to do.

There are other ways for mercury amalgam to find itself in trash.

Instruments used to place amalgam are rinsed or wiped off to remove leftover filling particles prior to sterilization. The wipes used for this can end up in the garbage. Particles and chunks of old amalgams being drilled out fly out of the patients' mouths on to the floor to be vacuumed by the cleaning service. Then the vacuum bags are thrown into the trash. The suction device held by the dental assistant has a removable trap to catch larger particles. When these traps are removed, their contents should be kept in an air-tight container for recycling or disposed of in a manner consistent with any hazardous waste, but they may find their way into the garbage.

It's not just the living that pollute the environment with dental mercury. The dearly departed pollute it as well.

C h a p t e r 5

Burning issues: pollution from the dead

There are no EPA mercury emission limits for crematoria.[354a]

Pacemakers are often removed before cremation to prevent the small amount of radioactive isotopes they contain from being released into the air. But until recently, no one has been overly concerned about the mercury amalgam fillings vaporizing during cremation. In a 1990 study conducted in England, it was calculated that the typical crematorium would release 24 pounds of mercury per year from fillings.[355]

According to the Cremation Association of North America, the number of crematories in the U. S. in 1993 was 1,058. The projected number of crematories in the U.S. for the year 2010 is about 1260. The number of cases per crematory in the U.S. for 1993 was 423.9. The projected number of cases per crematory in the U.S. in the year 2010 will sharply increase to 677.5. So the total number of cremations in the U.S. in 1993 was 448,500. And the projected total for U.S. cremations in the year 2010 is 853,500, almost double that of 1993.[355a]

If we assume that the typical crematorium in the U.S. also released 24 pounds of mercury in 1993, then by the year 2010 the typical U.S. crematory will be releasing 38.3 lbs per year based on the projected increase of cases per crematory. Using the same figures, if the yearly total mercury release from cremation in 1993 for the U.S. was 25,392 pounds then that will balloon to 47,880 pounds by the year 2010.

Pollution caused by mercury fillings doesn't stop after one dies. The dead can inadvertently pollute the living during cremation. Mercury in the air is bad because it moves with the wind far from the source. Pristine areas far away can end up with the mercury rain. And the more mercury that winds up in the water, the less the fish can be eaten. Food sources become polluted, through soil and water contamination far from the pollution source.

Let's describe a scenario using a fictitious character, Bernie Ash, as an example of pollution from cremation. Our friend Bernie worked as an environmental consultant for air and water pollution. When he made his burial decisions, Bernie chose cremation over embalming because he thought it made more sense for the environment. Ashes, he knew, would provide fertilizer to spread around his roses.

Embalming made no sense to him, at all. He thought, "why preserve my body with poisonous formaldehyde"? He certainly didn't need it anymore and he was big on recycling. Bernie also preferred to save the resources and expenses required to manufacture the casket and vault.

One thing Bernie did want was a recycled plastic headstone placed under his favorite tree which read:

"Bernie Ash,
Here I am scattered.
I have become part of this tree;
I give you shade.
I am part of the rose you hold in your hand;
I give you beauty.
My body has returned to the ocean of atoms;
I am in and around all life."

Our buddy Bernie, just like most people, went to the dentist regularly and had "silver" amalgams in his teeth. Someone told him, however, just before he passed away, that he had mercury in his "silver" fillings. He was amazed. If his dentist had told him that his fillings were mostly mercury, he would not have had them placed in his cavities. Because of his environmental training, he was well aware of mercury's poisonous nature. He wondered to what extent his own disease was hastened by the mercury leaching from his amalgams, as he knew mercury can suppress the immune system.

203

Bernie found out that there were no mercury emission requirements for crematoria. He was appalled that the dental mercury going
into the atmosphere from crematoria would come down in rain
somewhere else, causing pollution both close and far away. So he
specifically requested in his will that his mercury fillings be removed
and disposed of as hazardous waste under the EPA guidelines. He
knew that outside his mouth, amalgams were considered hazardous
waste. His amalgams were removed and disposed of properly.
Unfortunately, he died before he had a chance to complete his campaign for mandatory amalgam removal prior to cremation. The
motto he picked for this movement was: "Rest easy, don't let your
'death poison the living."

Bernie had the good health of all of us in mind. While people are
alive, they can choose to have their mercury fillings removed before
cremation, to protect the environment. Then the burden of decision-
making in time of grief would be lessened for those left behind.

This decision, of course, will not have to be considered once dentistry becomes mercury-free.

The politics of amalgam

We have seen how amalgam has no place in the environment.
But are political and economic concerns ahead of health concerns?
All too often our priorities in this country seem to be in this order. If
we change our focus to health, the economic benefits will follow anyway. With good health, it costs much less in the long run through
savings in sickness and disease treatment. And, if we don't create a
health hazard in the beginning, we won't have to fix it later.

Are dentists still being told mercury amalgam fillings are safe
because the "power brokers" in dentistry have political and economic
agendas? There is overwhelming evidence demonstrating the adverse
health effects of dental amalgam, so why isn't something being done
about it?

1. Many dentists don't want to change to the new composite fillings because they cost the dentist more.

It also takes more skill and time to correctly place a good composite filling than it does a mercury-releasing amalgam. Because they are cheaper and take less skill and time to place, mercury fillings are more profitable to the dentist. However, if most dentists used composites, the increased purchasing volume would drive composite prices down.

Considering profit before health is bottom-line thinking. Too often I've seen bottom-line thinking take precedent over what is best for all of us. I believe a health professional can never go wrong setting the patient's best health as the first priority. Patients are getting more astute and often know if they are at a bottom-line, profit-centered office or a health-centered office.

2. Insurance companies don't want the floodgates of liability to open and wash away their profits.

What if the ADA admitted publicly that mercury from dental fillings can cause psychological, behavioral and learning disabilities as well as arthritis, MS-like symptoms and a whole host of other more dramatic nerve disorders and birth defects? Law schools might have to include a new course entitled "Dental Mercury Amalgam Law." The dental law business would be brisk.

3. The ADA uses the fear of increased dental costs to keep the consumer from seeing the true choice: safe vs. not safe.

Fortunately, the increase in composite filling cost over amalgam is not that great. According to *Dental Economics* May 1995, the national average fee for a one surface amalgam filling is $51. The national average for a one surface composite filling varies from $63 to $70 depending on its location in front teeth or back teeth.[355b] Would you pay $12 to $19 more for a filling you knew has no mercury in it or do you want to save $12 to $19 on the chance that symptoms of mercury poisoning won't appear in you right away?

We are at a crossroads. We have an opportunity to do it right from now on. We can choose to ban mercury in dentistry. The strength of our future and the future of our country, indeed our planet, depends on wise choices being made today. As you'll see, some European countries have already made wise choices to protect people's health.

Amalgam banned in other countries

On February 18, 1994, the Swedish government banned mercury/silver amalgam as a dental filling material. Hooray! The ban was based on research demonstrating that the risks to dental patients' health and the risks to the environment are too great.[356] Despite the research being freely available, the United States government and the ADA have chosen to continue using mercury amalgam in the United States.

In February 1992, the German Federal Department of Health banned the sale and manufacture of one type of amalgam because of the health risks from mercury. A second type was restricted a short time later. The U.S. has not restricted amalgam use at all.

In December 1993, the largest manufacturer of dental amalgam in Germany discontinued production of amalgam. I surmise they wanted to limit their liability. So far, the powers that exist in the U.S. don't see the same picture. I believe that when the question of liability finally arises in the U.S., there will be a lot of fast and furious changes. The number of legal issues may be limited by the ADA or the government if mercury amalgams are banned sooner rather than later. There is no question in my mind or the minds of thousands of other professionals and lay persons that a ban is inevitable.

Early in 1994, the German Federal Department of Health advised against using amalgam in all women of childbearing age. Later, the German Federal Registry of Dentists requested that amalgam be banned. It did so because recent cases against a dental materials producer and the warning from the Department of Health left dentists legally liable for using mercury.[357]

Austria, Denmark and Finland plan dental mercury ban

Austria, Denmark and Finland have all said they plan to stop the use of mercury amalgam by the year 2000.[358] Why is the United States not among the countries acting on this important health issue? Other countries have already reviewed and evaluated the health risks of dental mercury and they have moved to eliminate those risks for their people and our environment.

Warning labels required on amalgam in California

As a result of a lawsuit, one of the largest dental amalgam manufacturers in the United States was ordered to place warning labels on amalgam packaging and provide warning signs to be posted in dental offices. The labels were to inform patients that exposure to mercury may cause birth defects and miscarriages. The warning signs read:

"This office uses amalgam filling materials which contain and expose you to mercury, a chemical known to the State of California to cause birth defects and other reproductive harm. Please consult your dentist for more information." [359]

How can California know that mercury causes birth defects and require warning labels on amalgam packages, while the rest of the United States does nothing? I was proud to see California taking this bold and important first step to protect public health. California was the first state to have strong consumer pressure. The difference in how amalgam lives or dies in a state or country lies in the ability of the government to heed consumers' wishes and the strength of those wishes. One voice is the beginning of a choir; don't hesitate to sing out.

Unfortunately, this consumer victory in California was short-lived. The heavy hand of industry slammed the door on warning the consumer about mercury amalgam. In August 1994, a federal judge in San Diego, California, ruled in favor of the dental amalgam manufacturers, saying that dentists and amalgam manufacturers do not have to comply with Proposition 65, passed by voters in 1986. Proposition 65 required consumers be warned about products containing potentially harmful compounds.

Attorney Carol Brophy, representative of the Committee of Dental Amalgam Alloy Manufacturers and Distributors, said that the country's manufacturers of medical devices can now "rest easy."[360] The score is business 2, consumers 1, but this game is not over.

More good news; water being cleaned up

Two apparently safe and effective means of mercury clean up in water have been discovered recently.

The first success story involves Sweden's use of selenium blocks lowered into polluted lakes. These blocks have significantly reduced mercury levels in the 300 lakes where fishing is banned. They work by attracting mercury and pulling it out of the water. Mercury "sticks" to the selenium. Maybe water recycling or treatment plants could use this technology to reduce water pollution.

The second means of cleanup involves the use of two bacteria, *desulfo vibrio* and *desulfo maculum*. Ron Cohen, professor of environmental science at the Colorado School of Mines, said these little bugs can remove better than 99 percent of mercury, lead, cadmium and zinc from polluted rivers and streams. Could wastewater treatment or recycling plants use these bugs, too?[361]

Yes, mercury has done harm in our bodies and to our planet. Now is the right time to seek ways to reverse our indiscretions. Advances in technology have been increasingly directed at pollution control and the sustainable use of resources, and it has become front page news. As our population grows, the pressure we generate on our planet increases daily, and solutions to our growing impact are being discovered through foresight and vision.

As a result, we have newer, safer products to replace outdated and dangerous materials. I understand that composite resin fillings arose as an offspring of technologies developed for our aerospace industry. These fillings have proven themselves superior to mercury amalgam in laboratories and in the mouth. We have the ability to do so many things better, including dental fillings. Let's do it.

What can I really do?

Many people ask me what they can do. Some feel that the mercury problem may be so big, nothing they do would have an impact. Just the opposite is true. Everything you do has an impact.

> You can do something about mercury in the water.
> You can do something about mercury in fish.
> You can do something about mercury in the soil.
> You can do something about mercury in solid waste.
> You can do something about mercury in the air.
> You can do something about mercury in incinerators.
> You can do something about mercury in crematoria.

You can do something about mercury simply by telling your dentist you want him or her to use the newer, safer, better looking and longer lasting composites instead of the toxic, unsafe, mercury-containing and mercury-releasing amalgams.

Chapter 5

6

safe, strong

& healthy

Our Future
Is Now

Safe, Strong and Healthy

This chapter reviews the previous chapters and includes thoughts I have regarding our future health. It provides practical considerations to those choosing to be mercury-free. And the concluding pages elaborate my philosophy of practice and thoughts on a healthier future for ourselves, our children and our planet.

Our future is now

I believe an inquiring mind and the ability to change are two wise and noble attributes. If we stop learning, we become history. If we continue learning, we become the future.

We create the future every second of every minute of every day.

We can decide to make it healthy. A healthy future depends on three things: our food, our thoughts and our actions. Food, thought and actions can make us sick, or make us well. I speak of these three as if they are separate only for ease of discussion, as no part is truly separate from the whole. For example, there is food for our body and food for thought. There is action created by thought and thought-provoking action. And thinking about food usually initiates action.

This wholeness, or synergism, exists in our larger body, the Earth. What we do with the Earth can either enhance or hinder our well-being. I believe that all events, large and small have significance. The smallest thing may be most significant. For example, one may feel it is fine to throw trash out of a moving car, but if everyone felt the same, we'd be knee deep in garbage on our city streets and highways. I encourage you to keep in mind the impact your decisions may have on others and our environment. What is best for you is very often best for others and our planet.

A dental amalgam is small, but it has a measurable impact on human health. Amalgam also has environmental consequences which affect our health. And if one adds up the number of amalgams placed in the U.S. in just one year, 100 million, that one small filling becomes part of a very large problem. The greatest source of mercury exposure to Americans is dental fillings. The best way to stop the problem is through consumer education. The dental consumer can then make an informed choice about mercury fillings. I have confidence that the healthy choice will be made.

Let's quickly go over what we've learned in this book so far, chapter by chapter.

I Wanted to Graduate

In the first chapter I relate how I became aware of the dental mercury issue. Dental school taught me nothing about mercury amalgam's toxicity, allergenicity, environmental hazards or bioelec-

213

tromagnetic problems. The professors merely answered my questions on amalgam with, "When mercury is mixed with the silver powder its toxic properties are made harmless." This is the same misinformation fed to dentists by the American Dental Association. What I learned about mercury and its properties, I learned on my own. Dentists-in-training and dentists-in-practice are kept in the dark about mercury's negative health effects either by design or by neglect. What they should be taught is that there is no valid reason for dental mercury's continued use.

From Sickness to Health

The second chapter contains personal letters from a few of the thousands across the globe who have become mercury-free. They have led themselves from sickness to health. Often their sicknesses were labeled "non-curable" or "non-treatable" or "cause unknown." So many of these diseases with unknown causes abound in medical textbooks that it behooves the medical professions to seriously look at recovery stories such as those in this chapter. These marvelous testimonies about improved qualities of life are being repeated across the world as more people become mercury-free. This is a chapter filled with hope; hope that many others with similar symptoms may also find some welcome relief; hope that by reading these testimonies, even more people may lead themselves from sickness to health.

Twinbirth -- Amalgam and the ADA

"Twinbirth -- Amalgam and the ADA" told why dentists began using amalgam. It also detailed how the history of amalgam and the history of the ADA are inextricably linked. Mercury was known to be poisonous before 1834, the year amalgam was introduced in the U.S. That is why over 150 years ago, the physicians who were also practicing dentists declared that mercury amalgam use was malpractice. But consumers wanted a painless filling and they found it in amalgam. As a result, the demand for amalgam quickly grew. Convenience, profitability and ignorance fueled the market for mercury fillings. Medical concerns were swept aside in the tidal wave of patients' demands.

Today the tide is changing direction. Dental mercury is no better than it was in 1834. But we have an improved understanding of mercury's interaction with living systems. And our technological advances have given birth to an entire family of alternative filling materials. Stronger, safer and more attractive filling materials, coupled with scientific evidence of mercury's harm, demand that medical concerns about mercury become a priority once again.

Mercury-A Universe of Trouble

The fourth chapter relates the far-reaching havoc mercury can wreak on our bodies and personalities. Over 200 symptoms of mercury poisoning are listed in the scientific and medical literature. Mercury affects every single system in the body. From anxiety to mood swings, from irritability to memory loss, mercury interferes with happiness and balance. From the brain to the kidneys and the mouth to the heart, mercury chokes and clogs the machinery of healthy living. Arthritis-like pain, Multiple Sclerosis-like symptoms, chronic fatigue, behavioral changes, insulin inhibition, immune suppression and death all describe destructive pathways mercury may take through the human body.

Mercury on Earth

"Mercury on Earth" explores mercury's widespread contamination of our planet, some of which happened years ago, some today. Both dental mercury and mercury from other sources pollute our world. However, the World Health Organization and mercury

215

experts agree that dental mercury amalgam is by far the largest source of mercury exposure in the general population.[362,363]

Large scale tragedies have followed mercury's poisoning of the soil, water and air. Our Everglades National Park is heavily polluted with mercury which concentrates in the food chain. Scientists fear the world's worst mercury-induced environmental disaster is unfolding in the jungles of Brazil. And a large portion of the disaster is caused by dental mercury.

Small scale tragedies are no less painful personally, and have spurred legislation to ban mercury in interior and exterior latex paint in the United States. Mercury has also been banned in many pesticides in America. But mercury is still allowed in the most personal environment of the mouth. I wonder who has the most powerful lobby in Washington: the paint industry, pesticide industry or the ADA?

Mercury from dental amalgam was found to have caused large areas of contamination in Connecticut soil. As a result, the state EPA declared amalgam a hazardous substance under the Superfund law. It is ludicrous to believe that amalgam in the backyard is hazardous but in a person's mouth it's fine. Yet, that is what we are being told.

Mercury from dental amalgam contaminates wastewater coming from dental offices. There are no standard limits for mercury content in wastewater and no routine testing of wastewater to determine mercury sources or levels.

Mercury from dental amalgam poisons our air. Leftover pieces of amalgam may get thrown out with the trash and end up in a solid waste incinerator. When heated, amalgam releases large quantities of mercury into the atmosphere. Most mercury emissions into the air, in fact, come from solid waste incinerators. Another hidden way for mercury from dental fillings to enter the air we breathe is from crematoria, which have no mercury emission requirements. The mercury vapor from amalgam may travel great distances and be deposited in high mountains and pristine wilderness areas far from the polluting source.

Logically then, if the use of mercury decreases, the possibility for contamination decreases. It seems that much environmental degradation could be avoided with the use of mercury-free fillings.

The dental office

Dental offices using amalgam can be highly contaminated with mercury vapor. Even offices that don't use amalgam now, but used it in the past, may also be contaminated. Carpeting in treatment rooms is impossible to clean after a mercury spill. And mercury vapor, once released, is circulated in all the common heating and air conditioning systems. If the dental office using amalgam is sharing space with a medical office, sick patients waiting for the physician may unknowingly breathe mercury vapor.

And what about the unsuspecting dentist and his or her staff? Most dentists and dental staff have absolutely no idea to what extent they are being exposed to mercury vapor from dental amalgam. Mercury vapor is completely undetectable by human senses. It has no taste or smell and is invisible. The first symptoms of mercury poisoning are subtle; symptoms such as anxiety, depression and mood swings. We can protect our valuable dental professionals by choosing mercury-free dentistry.

Now that I've jogged your memory about some of the major points of this book, I ask you to keep them in mind as I give you some final thoughts on dentists, dentistry, health and the power of the people.

Strength, thirst and hope

Rachel Carson's book, <u>Silent Spring</u>, taught us a great deal about personal power. She wrote her book about DDT and its threat to our health and our planet. But she also wrote her book about strength, thirst and hope. Carson had a thirst for truth, even though the truth ran contrary to what big business was telling us. She had the strength to write what turned out to be a classic book on environmental issues. And she had hope in us; hope that we, through reading her book, would change the way things were done. We rose to the challenge and gave life to her hope.

As a result of her book, DDT was banned. This one book put the word ecology into America's vocabulary and showed what strength of purpose can accomplish. Rachel Carson demonstrated that thirst for the truth supersedes profit and ignorance. She showed us there is always hope for our children's future. She showed us how beliefs shared by many can create momentum for positive change.

I am certain that just as DDT was banned through thirst, hope and strength, so will dental amalgam. We changed history when we banned DDT and we will change history again.

Why is mercury still used in fillings?

I believe most dentists are honest, hard-working and dedicated professionals who always attempt to do what they feel is best. However, for a professional to determine what is best, he or she must first have knowledge. If the information given to dentists is incomplete and unbalanced, then their decisions may suffer.

One reason most dentists still use mercury is lack of information. Dentists are not taught much, if anything, about mercury toxicity in dental school. And they don't hear much negative information on mercury amalgam from the pro-amalgam ADA. The result is that most dentists are underinformed in this area.

A second reason for the continued use of mercury fillings is resistance to change. I have heard ADA members paraphrase a favorite line of the ADA, "We've always done it this way. Amalgam has been used for 160 years and that fact alone is testimony to its safety." Do you really want a dentist to use technology developed over 160 years ago just because it has always been done that way? Leeches and bleedings were used for over 150 years in medicine, but that doesn't make those practices healthy or safe either.

The ADA has a responsibility to patients and the profession to disseminate accurate information. It has access to all the information on mercury, yet chooses to remain pro-amalgam. I believe that greed, an unwillingness to change, fear of litigation and fear of reduced political influence (power loss) are the factors largely shaping the ADA's opinion on the mercury issue.

Whole dentistry

Today there is an opportunity to move to a new level of dentistry. We realize our bodies are whole, not a bunch of parts installed together that need to be worked on piecemeal. This is what holistic healthcare is based upon. This includes the mind-body interactions each of us have. For example, we can make ourselves sick by worrying or we can speed our recovery by having a positive mental attitude. Emerging changes in holistic or mind-body living are being led by outstanding professionals such as Dr. Deepak Chopra, Dr. Dean Ornish, Dr. Bernie Segel and others. They point out the wholeness of our lives and the connections we have to our beliefs, each other, our Earth and the universe. The wholeness of dentistry can be achieved by expanding our awareness beyond teeth and tongues.

Environmental awareness is becoming more commonly included in personal philosophy for healthy living. More people understand that we live because the Earth lives. Without the Earth, we don't exist. Our health depends on the Earth's health. This new level of thinking for dentistry includes doing our best for our health as well as the Earth's. What we do individually affects the whole picture of living and health. Being mindful of these interconnections in the practice of dentistry is what I call whole dentistry.

Chapter 6

Health is happiness

I see personal health from a larger perspective than I did in the past. Anything that drains energy or creates stress (chemical, emotional, or physical), takes away some of a person's ability to achieve a sense of balance, a sense of well-being. Mercury fillings, which continually release poison into the body and have an unnatural electrical "fingerprint," create stress.

Conversely, anything that increases energy or removes blocks to feeling well can increase a sense of peace, tranquility and well-being. This can be achieved by a more healthful and balanced way of eating, eliminating exposure to a proven poison (like you-know-what), exercising and maintaining a positive mental outlook. Any one of these changes will increase well-being and happiness, but together they are very powerful.

Health is not just a condition of the body, it is also a state of mind. We can think ourselves sick. We can think ourselves well. Happiness is inextricably linked to health and vice versa. That is why I often say health is happiness. A choice to be healthy is a choice for happiness. Choosing composites over amalgam is a choice for health.

What and how we eat determines, to a large extent, how we feel and act. Food is the largest material factor in determining longevity and health. Our ability to chew greatly influences how much nourishment is extracted from each bite. What we chew our food on determines how wholesome and nutritious our food really is.

Clean food, clean fillings

Two important factors in good health are clean food and clean fillings. You wouldn't think of eating off a laboratory bench contaminated with mercury, yet chewing food on amalgam fillings contaminates the food with mercury just as surely as if you ate off that bench.

When you wrote on the sidewalk with chalk when you were young, remember how the chalk wore down? Well, the friction of chewing on mercury fillings does the same thing microscopically. Chewing on amalgam leaves a little mercury in every bite like chalk leaves a mark on the sidewalk. Mercury is the more poisonous twin of lead. Lead has been removed from gasoline, ceramic glazes and paint because of health concerns. You wouldn't dream of using a food processor that had blades made from 50% lead. Yet if you have mercury amalgams, you chop, cut and grind all your food on fillings that are 50% mercury. Teeth are our ultimate personal food processors. Chef yo! We slice, we dice, we make julienne fries in seconds! Mercury-free teeth give us mercury-free food.

Rather than purchase heavily processed or pesticide, herbicide, hormone or antibiotic-tainted food, many people choose to spend a little more for "clean" organic and minimally-processed food. Your priorities can be the same for "clean" composite fillings. It is better to spend money on sickness prevention rather than sickness treatment. Prevention is always less costly financially and emotionally. Mercury-free fillings can be part of your health maintenance plan.

Clean food is that much more important to children because their bodies are still under construction. You wouldn't use wood that was weakened with termites to build or repair a house. Why would you use food contaminated by mercury to build a child's body? Most parents, once they know of the dangers posed by mercury, want mercury-free fillings for their children.

Mercury build-up

That little bit of mercury added to food each time you chew can accumulate in the body over the years. It's kind of like waxy buildup on your kitchen floor. The first few times you wax, you can't see the build up, but a few layers later, the accumulation begins to be visible.

221

Mercury builds up when it trickles out of fillings into the body every second, every hour, every day of your life. You may feel fine for 20 years, then suddenly develop tiny, barely noticeable symptoms. A little depression here, a little arthritis there, fatigue and forgetfulness; you think "Ah, I'm just getting older." How many people would suspect their dental fillings as the cause of these problems? You may not have had a new filling put in for 20 years. Why should the old ones give you trouble now?

Everyone has different limits before the body rebels and says, "ENOUGH!" How much mercury can you take before you show adverse symptoms? The question is, "Why chew my food on a known poison?"

When you become mercury-free, your body may begin to clear its stored mercury. If the damage done by the stored mercury is not permanent, symptoms you may have as a result of mercury could lessen or disappear.

Your body, your garden

What happens to a garden that has been chemically fertilized for years vs. a garden that has only had organic mulch turned into the soil? Eventually, the chemical garden becomes out of balance (so one just adds more chemicals?). The organically mulched soil not only stays in balance, but becomes richer. Your body is your garden. Give it the best soil so your life stays in balance and becomes richer with the years. Keep chemicals like mercury out!

Question authority

We are creating an increasingly complex world. Our technological achievements have often outpaced our understanding of them -- biologically, emotionally and environmentally. Re-evaluating products and techniques is vital to our health and crucial to sustaining our resources. Accepting the status quo is business-as-usual. Questions must be directed to existing power structures, like the ADA and answers like, "Well, we've done it this way for years," are no longer acceptable. Those who listen and attempt to find answers will lead us into the light of the future, away from the dark ignorance of the past. You and I are the forces that create change when we ask questions and don't settle for hollow answers.

The phrase I remember so well from the 1960s was "Question Authority." When put into practice, it was the best catalyst for change. It still is. And I believe practicing this right is an obligation to ourselves and to our future generations. We deserve no less. Our future deserves our best.

Becoming mercury-free

If you wish to know more about becoming mercury-free, the next several pages will assist you. As each of us is unique, with our own set of circumstances, it is always wise to consult your primary care physician before deciding how best to proceed.

Replacing amalgams

So you have amalgams and want them replaced? Perhaps you're wondering what to do? Most people fall into one of two major categories: Those who are healthy and those who face health challenges. Those who are not in the best health need to be protected more closely from the temporary high mercury vapor levels generated by the dental drill during the removal process. Methods of protection are discussed below. But first, you must find a good dentist.

Finding a good dentist

I recommend you find a dentist who is mercury-free and who has a good reputation with health-conscious groups in your area. A true mercury-free dentist does not use mercury at all in the office. There are dentists in my area advertising that they are mercury-free, but they also place mercury fillings. So ask the dentist if he or she uses mercury at all in the office. Why? There may be mercury lingering in the office from the last patient who had three amalgams placed. Just as in other professions, there are dentists who perform with care and commitment. Unfortunately, there are also those who do mercury-free dentistry for less-than-altruistic reasons.

Just because a dentist claims to be mercury-free, don't assume that he or she is good. Ask friends. Ask the locals at the health food store. Ask alternative care physicians. Composite resins require more time and talent to install than amalgam. They can be more difficult to do well. You want to find a dentist who has talent, knowledge and a reputation for truly caring about you. Skill in placing composite restorations can be enhanced by years of use.

Amalgam replacement for healthy people

Let's say you decide to have your amalgams replaced and you have no health challenges. First of all, let me congratulate you on a wise choice for yourself and our planet! The benefits will remain with us beyond your lifetime. There are two ways you can approach replacement. The first is to set a goal for when you wish to be mercury-free and discuss it with your dentist. The second is to replace amalgams as they wear out and slowly, but eventually, become mercury-free.

Amalgam replacement for health-challenged people

It may be more important to people facing health problems to consider removing this toxin from their bodies sooner rather than later. That decision is best made by a physician familiar and qualified to review your individual medical needs. The longer the body is subjected to mercury vapor, the greater the amount of mercury that can lodge in vital organs and undermine health. However, each case must be reviewed on its own merit.

There are instances when amalgams should not be disturbed. For example, when a person is in the last stages of a terminal illness, it makes no sense to subject him or her to stressful dental procedures. The most important support for these people in transition is comfort and love. It is always wise to consult your physician before mercury amalgam removal.

Tests for mercury exposure

Tests to determine mercury exposure are best handled by those in the medical community who are qualified and able to conduct the proper tests. This means someone other than your dentist. The dentist's job is to provide answers to questions on mercury, remove the source of mercury exposure when the patient requests it and be available for followup care if needed.

Tests to determine mercury exposure are not needed unless there is a medical reason or you want to get a general idea of your exposure level. The problem with these tests are that none are 100% accurate. Accurate test results are complicated by differing forms of mercury as well as difficulty in detecting the low levels of mercury arising from dental amalgam. Mercury also vaporizes easily and can be lost from the test sample before the analysis is complete. I am most concerned about how much mercury is in the body and exposure tests do not reveal this.

I believe the real problem for most people with dental amalgam lies not in the quantity of mercury found on some test, but the length of time one has been exposed. As a result, I seldom recommend testing for mercury exposure. However, if you decide to be tested, I recommend seeking advice from a knowledgeable and qualified health-

225

care provider about the types of mercury testing available. Immunologists, toxicologists, allergy specialists and other professionals can be of help. Here are some common tests performed for mercury exposure:

Fecal analysis

This may be the most accurate technique for determining mercury vapor exposure. However, few labs do such tests and low-level chronic exposure such as that from dental amalgam is difficult to detect.

Hair analysis

Hair analysis to determine mercury exposure may be accurate for organic mercury but can vary in its accuracy with mercury vapor.[364] So it may be of limited value to the dental patient.

Urine and blood analysis

Neither of these tests are reliable enough to be used for low-level chronic mercury vapor exposure (the main type of exposure from amalgam).

Patch testing on the skin

There are a number of studies which suggest patch testing may have many false positive results. On the whole, it seems unreliable.

Mercury vapor measurements in the mouth

This is an excellent way to measure the amount of mercury

released from amalgam fillings. Potential tissue mercury levels may then be estimated.[365]

Precautions during mercury amalgam removal

During mercury amalgam removal the level of mercury vapor rises in and around the mouth due to the heat and increased amalgam surface area generated by the drill. Here are some methods available to reduce the mercury vapor exposure during the removal process:

1. Alternative air supply for patient provided through a nasal mask
2. Outside fresh air exchange for the office
3. Ionizing air filters in treatment rooms
4. High volume suction used in the mouth
5. High-speed drill with water spray and a diamond bur (drill bit)
6. Sectioning the fillings and removing them in pieces
7. A rubber dam to isolate the teeth from the mouth
8. Eye protection during drilling (mandatory)
9. Patient drape to cover clothing

Any of these precautions are helpful, but not all are possible or warranted every time. Each case must be evaluated individually. The precautions decided upon must take into consideration the entire health status of the patient. A thorough medical and dental history along with a complete dental examination gives the dentist a solid basis upon which to proceed. I again encourage those considering mercury amalgam removal to seek out a knowledgeable and caring professional.

What is sequential removal?

Sequential removal of amalgam means taking fillings out in a certain order based on their electrical qualities.

Because my father was an electronics engineer, I have a particular fondness for electrical knowledge. I believe that the most overlooked and least understood aspects of dental metals such as amalgam are their electrical qualities.

There has been a lot written about sequential removal. Complex theories based on electrical current measurements are not valid. This type of measurement inside the mouth is completely unreproducable and, therefore, unscientific and unreliable.

Voltage measurements, on the other hand, are reproducible and reliable. If you decide you want electrical testing done on the amalgams, make sure the test is to measure voltage, not current. If sequential removal is then desirable, the fillings with the largest voltage differences from natural tooth structure should be removed first. Simply put, the fillings with the greatest electrical differences from the body's natural voltages may present the greatest problems.

Mercury amalgams can cause electrical imbalances within the body and some patients need sequential removal of amalgams so as to not temporarily exacerbate their symptoms. But not all patients exhibit an amalgam-caused electrical imbalance. Even though some mercury-free advocates say everyone needs sequential removal, I have yet to see convincing proof of this.

Who needs sequential removal?

I have found that sequential removal of amalgam seems necessary when unexplained symptoms exist that may be caused by electrical interferences. Those symptoms include unexplained psychological or behavioral abnormalities, neurologic difficulties, especially around the head and neck region, ringing in the ears, hearing problems, vision disturbances, unexplained neuralgia or numbness or a metallic taste. It is always wise and in your best interest to make sure a physician has been consulted first about these kinds of symptoms. They may be medically, not dentally, based. If that is true, they may be indications of serious medical problems.

Sequential removal made easy

For two years, I measured the electrical potentials of every metal and every natural tooth in patients' mouths. I found that all amalgams followed the same pattern: The smaller the filling, the more electrically stimulating it could be, according to the voltage measurements. Nerves work on certain voltages. The small fillings' voltages had the greatest potential to stimulate nerves to fire. In other words, the worst electrically were the smallest. I suggest that the fillings that may act as nerve stimulants be taken out first. The ones acting like anesthetics should be taken out next. The last ones to be removed are the ones that are neutral to the nerve.

I have developed and used a rule of sequential removal for nearly 14 years with great success. If you need to have the amalgams taken out by sequential removal (electronic order) because of your symptoms, have them removed from smallest to largest. Remove the smallest amalgam first, and work upwards in size.

Four removal visits are typical to become mercury-free

Patients not needing sequential removal do fine by having amalgams removed in one quadrant (quarter) of the mouth at a time. Typically, four visits will complete amalgam removal for most healthy people.

Time between visits, how much and why?

It is important to take removal of mercury fillings at a pace which is not too fast. During the amalgam grinding process, you may be exposed to a brief high dose of mercury. This may exacerbate any existing symptoms resulting from mercury vapor exposure.

Generally, I have found that for most healthy persons a week to ten days between removal sessions is adequate. However, each case must be evaluated on how well each visit is tolerated. As much as two to three weeks between visits may be required in order to rid the body of any mercury burden that may have been added during the removal process.

Helping your body rid itself of mercury after each removal session is recommended in most cases. This is called mercury detoxification. There are a large number of effective medical and nutritional detoxification protocols.

Mercury detoxification

If you are following a detoxification regime -- and I recommend that you do -- your body will release mercury faster than if you just let nature take its course. Our bodies will naturally release stored mercury, but it can be a very slow process.

There are many different, valid and useful programs available. Consult your physician before going on a program, especially if you have medical problems or are on medication.

I encourage you to work with a physician, M.D., naturopath, homeopath, chiropractor or other healthcare provider who is knowledgeable and qualified in detoxifying the body from mercury.

What follows is a detox program which I recommend and use in coordination with my patients' primary care professionals.

As always, if you have a health challenge or are taking medication, check with your physician before beginning a detoxification program.

My four week mercury detoxification program includes:

First week:

Vitamin C, time released, 1000 mg twice a day
Vitamin A, 5,000 IU a day
Vitamin E, 200 IU a day
Vitamin B complex "for stress", 15 to 20 mgs of each B Vitamin,
   one a day
Zinc, chelated, 15-30 mg day
Manganese, 2.5-5 mg a day
Magnesium, 450 mg a day
Chromium, 0.2 mg a day

Second week:
decrease Vitamin C to 1500 mg a day, keep taking all others

Third week;:
decrease Vitamin C to 1000 mg a day
and decrease Vitamin A to 2500 IU a day, keep taking all others

Fourth week:
decrease Vitamin C to 500 mg a day, keep taking all others

You can stop the program at the end of the fourth week. If you schedule a removal session in the middle of the program, start it over as if it were the first week again.

I recommend you avoid sugar, carbonated beverages, caffeine, tobacco, alcohol, excessive dairy or meat products and processed foods.

Foods I recommend are complex carbohydrates, green salads, fresh or lightly steamed vegetables (especially asparagus), fresh fruit, eaten by itself and protein sources other than red meat.

If you are in excellent health, a good way to rid the body of mercury is in the steam room or sauna. The skin is the body's largest excretory organ. A good workout that makes you perspire is also effective. Be sure that you consult a physician before any of these sweat-producing eliminations are undertaken. Do not use megadoses of vitamins or minerals before consulting your physician.

How do composite fillings differ?

Composite fillings feel and look like normal teeth. They are invisible fillings. However, composite resins are much harder than amalgams. And their full hardness is achieved in seconds while you are in the dental chair. Amalgams take from a couple of days to several weeks to fully harden.

Because of their slow setting time, amalgams can be hammered into shape by the opposing teeth, flattening any high spots on the filling. As a result, very few adjustments on amalgams are required. However, since composites have a much higher initial strength, if they have any spots that hit the opposing teeth too soon, symptoms can arise. Indications of too-tall composites are: discomfort when chewing foods, especially with harder foods and temperature (usually more cold than hot) and/or flossing sensitivity.

The proper fit of composite fillings to the opposing teeth takes more time and care than amalgam fillings. Most patients are numb when their fillings are hardened, so the initial fit to the opposite teeth may not be perfect. All these problems can usually be eliminated with an additional adjustment of the new filling's chewing surface after the numbness has worn off.

The new composites will give you many years of excellent service and they'll make your teeth look like they have no fillings. I call it invisible dentistry. I presently have fillings made from the older generation composites that are almost 14 years old and they are still doing well.

Choosing the right composite

The right composite will not only give you gorgeous, invisible, mercury-free fillings, but will last a long time with proper care. Most people do well with any of the newer composite fillings. But on rare occasions, one might have an allergy to a composite. So the right composite may mean the strongest, or it may mean the most biocompatible with your body chemistry.

If you have a lot of allergies or are very sick, I suggest that you be tested by an allergist for composite material compatibility prior to amalgam removal. This would give you an idea of which dental materials may suit you best. Consult closely with an immunologist, toxicologist, allergist or other medical professional who is knowledgeable about dental material biocompatibilities.

Currently some of the best composites in terms of physical and clinical characteristics are:

> Herculite by Kerr
> P-50 by 3M
> Z-100 by 3M
> Conquest by Jeneric/Pentron
> Heliomolar RO by Ivoclar
> Ful-Fil by Caulk/Dentsply
> Isomolar by Ivoclar
> AH-1 by Kerr
> Heliomolar by Ivoclar and
> P-30 by 3M[366]

It is your right to request filling materials by name whenever you have fillings placed or replaced.

My intention with this book

My intention is and always has been to educate the dental consumer. I want to make a difference in the perception of health so that wise, knowledgeable choices may be made.

233

Chapter 6

The dental profession, to a large extent, is resisting the change from mercury to mercury-free dentistry. There is, however, so much to gain from this transition. Safer, stronger fillings, safer dental offices and a safer environment are the benefits of mercury-free dentistry. Every person's decision to be mercury-free affects all our lives positively.

I have but one voice, heard through this book. Let the dentists hear all your voices. They will listen. You pay for their salary, staff, office, car and house(s). In essence, you, the patients, are their employers. If you decide to not accept amalgam, it simply won't be used. I don't know where the phrase came from, but I love, "If the people lead, the leaders will follow." It is true.

Let us, as consumers, take a stand. Let us choose mercury-free dentistry, so that no more mercury can trickle out of dental fillings. Let us stop being human experiments. We can choose health and show courage where the ADA has failed. We can speak out for health, for all of us, our planet and our future.

It is your right to choose the best fillings.

It is your right to choose personal health.

It is your right to choose a safe environment.

In Health and Happiness.

POSTSCRIPT

If you are interested in furthur medical research findings supporting this book I suggest the following review article:

Lorsheider, F.L., Viing, M.J. and Summers, A.D. "Mercury Exposure from 'Silver' Tooth Fillings; Emerging Evidence Questions a Traditional Dental Paradigm." FASEB Journal Vol 9 pp 504-508, 1995

Federation of American Societies for Experimental Biology
9650 Rockville Pike - Bethesda, Maryland 20814-3998
Telephone: 301-530-7000 - FAX 301-530-7001
Internet Address: fasebinfo@faseb.org

BIBLIOGRAPHY

1. Phillips, R.W., Skinner's Science of Dental Materials, 7th Ed., W.B. Saunders Co., Phila, 1973

2. Meyer, Carl B., "Iowa Dental Board Suspends License",*International DAMS Newsletter*, Vol.IV:4 pp 10-11 Fall 1994

3. Hoffman-Axthelm, Walter, History of Dentistry, Quintessence Publishing Co., Inc. Chicago, 1981 p 292

4. *The Science of the Total Environment*, 99, 1990 p 23-35

5. Ross, W.D. and Sholiton, M.C., "Specificity of psychiatric manifestations in relation to neurotoxic chemicals", *Acta Phychiat Scand*, 67 suppl 303: 100-104, 1983

6. *JAMA* August 5, 1983

7. Utt, Harold D. "Mercury Breath... How Much Is Too Much?"*California Dental Assoc J* Feb. 1984 pp 41-45

8. *Journal of Orthomolecular Medicine*, Vol. 5, #2, 1990

9. *Psychological Reports*, 70, 1992, p1139-1151

10. U.S. Dept. of Labor, Occupational Safety and Health Administration, August 1975, Job Health Hazards Series, "Mercury" OSHA 2234

11. Federal Register, Vol. 47, No. 2 Tuesday, January 5, 1982, p 441

12. Physician's Desk Reference, 47th Ed., Medical Economics Data, Oradell, N.J., 1993

13. Taber's Cyclopedic Medical Dictionary, Ed. 17 F.A. Davis Co. Philadelphia 1993

14. Foulds, D., et al. "Mercury poisoning and acrodynia ", *Am J Dis Children* 141:124-125, 1987

15. Sexton, D., et al. "A nonoccupational outbreak of inorganic mercury vapor poisoning" *Arch Environ Health* 33:186-191, 1976

16. Bourgeois, M., et al. "Mercury intoxication after topical application of a metallic mercury ointment", *Dermatologica* 172:48-51 1986

17. "Mono That Lingers... For Years", *Th Harvard Medical School Health Letter* Vol.) No. 7, May 1985

18. Miller, N., "Vaccines and Natura Health", *Mothering*, No. 70:44-53, Sprin; 1994

19. Heidam, L.Z., "Spontaneous abortio amoung dental assistants, factory workers an gardening workers: a follow up study" *Epidemiol Commun Health*, 38:149-155, 198

20. Sikorski, R., et al. "Women in denta surgeries: Reproductive hazards in occupa tional exposure to mercury", *Int Arch Occu Environ Health*, 59:551-557, 1987

21. Guerini, V. ; A History of Dentistry Le and Febiger, Philadelphia and New York 1909, p 89

22. C. Plinius Secundus, The Natural Histor of Pliny translated by J. Bostock and H.T Riley, London, H.G. Bohn, 1857, Vol. 4 book 33

23. Weinberger, B.W.: An Introduction to th History of Dentistry in America. Vol. II St Louis, The C.V. Mosby Co., 1948

24. Weinberger, B.W.: An Introduction to th History of Dentistry in America. Vol. I St Louis, The C.V. Mosby Co., 1948, p 240

25. Greener, E.H."Amalgam-Yesterday,Today and Tomorrow" *Operative Dentistry* 4:24-3 1979

26. "George Washington, Medical Martyr" *Wellness Today*, Phillips Publishing, Potomac MD, Summer 1992

27. Harris, Chapin A.; The Principles anc Practice of Dental Surgery, Second Edition Lindsay and Blakiston, Philadelphia, 1845 p 259

28. Hine, M.K. Ed.; Review of Dentistry, Questions and Answers, Fifth ed. The C.V. Mosby Co. St. Louis, 1970

29. Wenig, Martin, "The rise of dentistry as a profession", Dental Students' Magazine Sept. 1943, p 16

30. Bremner, M.D.K. ; The Story of Dentistry, Dental Items of Interest Publishing Co. Inc., Brooklyn, N.Y. 1939, p 69

31. Harris, Chapin A.; The Principles and Practice of Dental Surgery, Second Edition, Lindsay and Blakiston, Philadelphia, 1845, p 252

32. Harris, Chapin A.; The Principles and Practice of Dental Surgery, Second Edition, Lindsay and Blakiston, Philadelphia, 1845, p 23

33. Hine, M.K. Ed.; Review of Dentistry, Questions and Answers, Fifth ed. The C.V. Mosby Co. St. Louis, 1970

34. Harris, Chapin A.; The Principles and Practice of Dental Surgery, Second Edition, Lindsay and Blakiston, Philadelphia, 1845, pp. 259-260

35. Ibid

36. Ibid

37. Ibid

38. Stillman, Paul R., "Progress in dentistry", Can Dent Assoc J Vol. IV, 1938

39. Levy, Morton J. "Gold Foil, Silver Amalgma, And Silicates--- Their Properties and Relative Merits" The Dental Student's Magazine , Nov. 1942 pp 21-25

40. Torres, H. O. and Ehrlich, A., Modern Dental Assisting, W.B. Saunders Co. Phila., PA 1980, p22

41. Harris, Chapin A.; The Principles and Practice of Dental Surgery, Second Edition, Lindsay and Blakiston, Philadelphia, 1845. p 24-25

42. Hine, M.K. Ed.; Review of Dentistry, Questions and Answers, Fifth ed. The C.V. Mosby Co. St. Louis, 1970

43. Harris, Chapin A.; The Principles and Practice of Dental Surgery, Second Edition, Lindsay and Blakiston, Philadelphia, 1845, p 25

44. Hine, M.K. Ed.; Review of Dentistry, Questions and Answers, Fifth ed. The C.V. Mosby Co. St. Louis, 1970

45. Bremner, M.D.K. ; The Story of Dentistry, Dental Items of Interest Publishing Co. Inc., Brooklyn, N.Y. 1939

46. Torres, H. O. and Ehrlich, A., Modern Dental Assisting, W.B. Saunders Co. Phila., PA 1980

47. Wenig, Martin, "The rise of dentistry as a profession", Dental Students' Magazine Sept. 1943, p 18

48. Bremner, M.D.K. ; The Story of Dentistry, Dental Items of Interest Publishing Co. Inc., Brooklyn N.Y. 1939, p 86-87

49. Ibid

50. Svare, C.W., et al, "Dental amalgam: a potential source of mercury vapor exposure", J Dent Res, 59 Special issue A: p 341, abstract 293, 1980

51. Svare, C.W., et al. "The effect of dental amalgams on mercury levels in expired air," J Dent Res 60:1668-1671, Sept. 1981

52. Reports of Councils and Bureaus "Significance to health of mercury used in dental practice: a review." JADA, Vol.82, June 1971 pp 1401-1407 Reprinted by permission of ADA Publishing Co., Inc.

53. Taylor, Joseph, Ed., ADA News, Vol. 15 January 2, 1984, p 4 Reprinted by permission of ADA Publishing Co., Inc.

54. Ibid

55. Interview with Dr. Lars Friberg by Tom Mangold in the Panorama production of "Poison in your Mouth" produced by the British Broadcasting Corporation, aired on July 11, 1994

56. Quote from Chris Martin of the ADA Communications Dept. (312) 440-2500 to Patricia Denninger August, 1994
57. Recommendations in mercury hygiene, 1984; *JADA* Vol. 109 Oct. 1984 pp 617-619 Reprinted by permission of ADA Publishing Co., Inc.
58. Ibid
59. Ibid
60. Ibid
61. Ibid
62. Reports of Councils and Bureaus "Significance to health of mercury used in dental practice: a review." *JADA*, Vol.82, June 1971 pp 1401-1407 Reprinted by permission of ADA Publishing Co., Inc.
63. Ibid
64. Recommendations in mercury hygiene, 1984; *JADA* Vol. 109 Oct. 1984 p617-619 Reprinted by permission of ADA Publishing Co., Inc.
65. Ibid
66. Ibid
67. Ibid
68. Ibid
68. "When Your Patients Ask About Dental Amalgam" (no author cited) *JADA* Vol. 122 No. 9 Aug. 1991 unnumbered tear-out page inserted in the *JADA* after page 80.
69. Recommendations in mercury hygiene, 1984; *JADA* Vol. 109 Oct. 1984 p617-619 Reprinted by permission of ADA Publishing Co., Inc.
70. Ibid
71. Ibid
72. Ibid
73. Ibid
74. Ibid
75. *Dentistry Today*, October, 1988 page 12
76. Clarkson, T.W., *New England Journal of Medicine* 323:1137-1139, Oct. 18,1990

Reprinted by permission Rochester University
77.WHO,1991, "Environmental Health Criteria 118: Inorganic Mercury", Geneva
78. Dr. Bernard P. Tillis' letter in Viewpoint, My View, "Doctor Heal Thyself" *ADA News,* Aug. 13, 1984 Re-printed by permission of ADA Publishing Co., Inc.
79. Dr. John W. Stamm, a dentist and epidemiologist, Dean of the School of Dentistry and chief of the Dental Research Center at the University of North Carolina, Chapel Hill, in the Special Report insert to the *JADA* , Jan. 1991
80. *CRA Newsletter* Vol. 18, Issue 5, May 1994
81. NIOSH A Recommended Standard for Occupational Exposure to Inorganic Mercury", U.S. Dept. of HEW Public Health Service 1977-757-009/42
82. Ibid
83. Ibid
84. Ibid
85. Ibid
86. Ibid
87. U.S. Dept. of Labor, Occupational Safety and Health Administration, August 1975, Job Health Hazards Series, "Mercury" OSHA 2234
88. Ibid
89. Phillips, Ralph W. Skinner's Science of Dental Materials, W.B. Saunders and Co. Philadelphia, 7th Ed. 1973 p 49-50
90. Ibid
91. Ibid p 519
92. Weiss, B., "Behavioral toxicology and environmental health science. Opportunity and challenge for psychology", *Am Psychologist,* Nov. 1983, pp 1174-1187
93. Queen, H.L., Chronic Mercury Toxicity, A new Hope Against an Endemic Disease, Queen and Co. Health communications,

Inc., Colorado Springs, Co., 1988, p17
94. Mercury, draft for public comment, United States Dept. of Health and Human Services, PHS, Oct. 1992, p 1
95. Utt, H. D., "Mercury breath... How much is too much?" *California Dental Association Journal,* Feb. 1984, pp 41-45
96. Svare, C.W., et al, "Dental amalgam : a potential source of mercury vapor exposure", *J Dent Res,* 59 Special issue A: p341, abstract 293, 1980
97. Mercury, draft for public comment, United States Dept. of Health and Human Services, PHS, Oct. 1992
98. Trakhtenberg, I.M., Chronic effects of mercury on organisms, US dept. of Health Education and Welfare, Public Health Service,National Institutes of Health. DHEW Pub. No. (NIH) 74-473, USGPO, Wash D.C., 1974
99. Vallee, B.L. and Ulmer, D.D., "Biochemical effects of mercury, cadmium and lead", *Ann Rev Biochem,* 41, 1972, pp 91-127
100. Robison, Steve H., et al, "Strand breakage and decreased molecular weight of DNA induced by specific metal compounds.", *Carcinogenesis,* 3(6):657-662, 1982
101. Matsuoka, Y. and Norden, B., "Effects of Ag+ and Hg2+ on the structure of DNA in solution studied by flow linear dichroism", *Biopolymers,* Vol. 22:601-604, 1983
102. Lehninger, A.L., Biochemistry, Worth Publishers, Inc., 1972
103. Menashi, et al., "Transplacental effects of methylmercury chloride in mice with specific emphasis on the audiogenic seizure response.", *Dev Neurosci,* 5:216-221, 1982
104. Tedeschi, L.G., "The Minamata disease", *Am J Forensic Med Pathol,* 3(4):335-

338, 1982
105. Harada, M., "Congenital Minamata disease: Intrauterine methylmercury poisoning." *Teratology,* 18(2):285-288, 1978
106. Queen, H.L., Chronic Mercury Toxicity, New Hope Against an Endemic Disease, Queen and Co. Health Communications, Inc. Colorado Sprgs, CO, 1988 p17-18
107. Elhassani, S.B., "The many faces of methylmercury poisoning", *J Toxicol.: Clin. Toxicol.,* 19(8):875-906, 1982-1983
108. Edwards, T., and McBride, B.C., "Nature", 253 (London), 1975, p.24
109. Rowland, I.R. and Grasso, P. and Davies, M. J., "The methylation of mercury chloride by human intestinal bacteria," *Experientia,* 31, 1975, pp 1064-1065
110. Heintze, U. et al, "Methylation of mercury from dental amalgam and mercuric chloride by oral streptococci in vitro", *Scand J Dent Res,* 91(2), 1983, pp150-152
111. Campbell, J., "Acute mercurial poisoning by inhalation of mercury vapor in an infant", *Can Med Assoc J* 58:72-75, 1948
112. Hallee, T.J.,"Diffuse lung disease caused by inhalation of mercury vapor", *Am Rev Respir Dis,* 99:430-436, 1969
113. Siblerud R.L. 1990 "The relationship between mercury from dental amalgam and the cardiovascular system. *Sci Total Environ* , 99(1-2):23-26
114. Piikivi, L., "Cardiovascular reflexes and low long-term exposure to mercury vapour", *Int Arch Environ Health,* 61(6):391-395, 1989
115. Trakhtenberg, I.M., Chronic effects of mercury on organisms, US dept. of Health Education and Welfare, Public Health Service,National Institutes of Health. DHEW Pub. No. (NIH) 74-473, USGPO, Wash D.C., 1974

239

116. Mercury, draft for public comment, United States Dept. of Health and Human Services, PHS Oct. 1992 p. 69
117. Karpathios et al, 1991 "Mercury vapor poisoning associated with hyperthyroidism in a child" *Acta Paediatr Scand* 80(5): 551-552
118. The Merck Manual of Diagnosis and Therapy, 16th Ed. R. Berkow, M.D. Ed., Merck Research Labs., N.J. 1992 p1080
119. The Merck Manual of Diagnosis and Therapy, 16th Ed. R. Berkow, M.D. Ed., Merck Research Labs., N.J. 1992 pp1057-1059
120. Trakhtenberg, I.M., Chronic effects of mercury on organisms, US dept. of Health Education and Welfare, Public Health Service,National Institutes of Health. DHEW Pub. No. (NIH) 74-473, USGPO, Wash D.C., 1974
121. Lehninger, A.L., Biochemistry, Worth Publishers, Inc., 1972
122. Tedeschi, L.G., "The Minamata disease", *Am J Forensic Med Pathol,* 3(4):335-338, 1982
123. Burton, B.V. and Meikle, A.W., "Acute and chronic methylmercury poisoning impairs rat adrenal and testicular function", *J Toxicol Environ Health,* 6:597-606, 1980
124. Hughes, J.A. and Annau, Z. "Postnatal behavioral effects in mice after prenatal exposure to methylmercury", *Pharmacol Biochem Behav* 4:385-391, 1976
125. Khera, K.S., "Teratogenic effects of methylmercury in the cat: note on the use of this species as a model for teratogenicity studies", *Teratology* 8:293-304, 1973a.
126. Lee, I.P., and Dixon, R.L., "Effects of mercury on spermatogenesis studies by velocity sedimentation cell separation and serial mating", *J Pharmacol Exp Ther* 194: 171-181, 1975
127. Mishonova, V.N., et al. "Characteristics of the course of pregnancy and births in women with occupational contact with small concentrations of metallic mercury vapors in industrial facilities", *Gig Truda Prof Zabol,* 24(2):21-23, 1980
128. Heidam, L.Z., "Spontaneous abortion amoung dental assistants, factory workers and gardening workers: a follow up study" *J Epidemiol Commun Health,* 38:149-155, 1984
129. Sikorski, R., et al. "Women in dental surgeries: Reproductive hazards in occupational exposure to mercury", *Int Arch Occup Environ Health,* 59:551-557, 1987
130. Derobert, L. and Tara,S., "[Mercury intoxication in pregnant women]" *Ann Med Leg,* 30:222-225, 1950
131. Cordier, S., et al., "Paternal exposure to mercury and spontaneous abortions" , *Br J ind Med* 48(6):375-381, 1991
132. Campbell, J., "Acute mercurial poisoning by inhalation of mercury vapor in an infant", *Can Med Assoc J* 58:72-75, 1948
133. Sexton, D., et al. "A nonoccupational outbreak of inorganic mercury vapor poisoning", *Arch Environ Health,* 33:186-191, 1976
134. *Mercury-Free News,* May 1992, p6
135. The Merck Manual of Diagnosis and Therapy, 16th Ed. R. Berkow, M.D. Ed., Merck Research Labs., N.J. 1992 pp 841-842
136. Taber's Cyclopedic Medical Dictionary, 17th Ed., C.L.Thomas M.D., M.P.H., Ed., F.A. Davis Co., PA, 1993 p 414
137. The Merck Manual of Diagnosis and Therapy, 16th Ed. R. Berkow, M.D. Ed., Merck Research Labs., N.J. 1992 p 2697
138. Ibid p 842
139. Svare, C.W., et al, "Dental amalgam: a potential source of mercury vapor exposure", *J Dent Res,* 59 Special issue A: p 341, abstract 293, 1980

140. The Merck Manual of Diagnosis and Therapy, 16th Ed. R. Berkow, M.D. Ed., Merck Research Labs., N.J. 1992 p 1310

141. The Merck Manual of Diagnosis and Therapy, 16th Ed. R. Berkow, M.D. Ed., Merck Research Labs., N.J. 1992, p 834

142. The Merck Manual of Diagnosis and Therapy, 16th Ed. R. Berkow, M.D. Ed., Merck Research Labs., N.J. 1992 p 830

143. Taber's Cyclopedic Medical Dictionary, 17th Ed., C.L.Thomas M.D., M.P.H., Ed., F.A. Davis Co., Philadelphia, 1993, p 239

144. Rothstein, A., "Mercurials and red cell membranes", Progress in Chemical and Biological Research, 51:105-131, 1981

145. Ibid

146. Verschaeve, L. et al. Genetic damage induced by occupationally low mercury exposure", Environ Res 12:306-316, 1976

147. Popescu, H.I., et al. "Chromosome aberrations induced by occupational exposure to mercury", Arch Environ Health, 34:461-463, 1979

148. Skerfving, S. et al. "Chromosome breakage in humans exposed to methylmercury through fish consumption", Arch Environ Health, 21:133-139, 1970

149. Skerfving, S. et al. "Methylmercury-induced chromosome damage in man", Environ Res, 7:83-98, 1974

150. Taber's Cyclopedic Medical Dictionary, 17th Ed., C.L.Thomas M.D., M.P.H., Ed., F.A. Davis Co., Philadelphia, 1993, p 1101

151. Taber's Cyclopedic Medical Dictionary, 17th Ed., C.L.Thomas M.D., M.P.H., Ed., F.A. Davis Co., Philadelphia, 1993 p 1306

152. Campbell, J., "Acute mercurial poisoning by inhalation of mercury vapor in an infant", Can Med Assoc J 58:72-75, 1948

153. Matthes, F., et al. "Acute poisoning associated with inhalation of mercury vapor: Report of four cases", Pediatrics, 22:675-688, 1958

154. Siblerud, R.L., "The relationship between mercury from dental amalgam and the cardiovascular system", Sci Total Environ, 99(1-2):23-36, 1990

155. Sarascia, M.M. et al., "Human Factor XIII - Metal Ion Interactions", J Biolg Chem, 257(23), 1982, pp 14102-14108

156. Leone, G., et al, "Human platelet aggregation by Thimerosal Functional and ultrastructural studies", Haemostasis, 8: 390-399, 1979

157. The Merck Manual of Diagnosis and Therapy, 16th Ed. R. Berkow, M.D. Ed., Merck Research Labs., N.J. 1992, p 1127

158. Mercury, draft for public comment, United States Dept. of Health and Human Services, PHS Oct. 1992, p 19

159. Jaffe, K.M., et al. "Survival after acute mercury vapor poisoning--the role of intensive supportive care", Am J Dis Child, 137:749-751, 1983

160. Taber's Cyclopedic Medical Dictionary, 17th Ed., C.L.Thomas M.D., M.P.H., Ed., F.A. Davis Co., Philadelphia, 1993 p 967

161. Ibid

162. Eggleston, D.W., "Effect of dental amalgams and nickel alloys on T-lymphocytes: Preliminary report", J Prosth Dent, 51(5):617-623, May 1984

163. Ibid

164. Ibid

165. Koller, L.S., "Immunotoxicology of heavy metals", Int J Immunopharmacol, 2:269-279, 1980

166. Taber's Cyclopedic Medical Dictionary, 17th Ed., C.L.Thomas M.D., M.P.H., Ed.,

F.A. Davis Co., Philadelphia, 1993 p 969
167. Moszczynski, P., et al. "The serum immunoglobulins in workers after prolonged occupational exposure to the mercury vapors" *Rev Roum Med Intern* 28(1):25-30, 1990b
168. Bencko, V., et al, "Immunological profiles in workers occupationally exposed to inorganic mercury", *J Hyg Epidemiol Microbiol Immunol* 34(1):9-15, 1990
169. Summers, A., et al. "Mercury released from dental 'silver' fillings provokes an increase in mercury- and antibiotic-resistant bacteria in oral and intestinal floras of primates", *Antimicrobial Agents and Chemotherapy*, 37(4): 825-834, Apr. 1993
170. "Amalgams May Be Suspect in Bacteria Resistance, Report's Findings Suggest" *Dentistry Today*, May 1993, p 20 Reprinted by permission of *Dentistry Today*
171. Ostlin, L. et al. "Amalgm removal - a road to better health?" Health Insurance Bureau, Stockholm County, Sweden, 1991
172. Taber's Cyclopedic Medical Dictionary, 17th Ed., C.L.Thomas M.D., M.P.H., Ed., F.A. Davis Co., Philadelphia, 1993, p 153-154
173. The Merck Manual of Diagnosis and Therapy, 16th Ed. R. Berkow, M.D. Ed., Merck Research Labs., N.J. 1992, p 1305
174. Theodore H. Ingalls, M.D., "Epidemiology, Etiology and prevention of multiple sclerosis. Hypothesis and Fact", *American Journal of Forensic Medicine and Pathology*, 4(1) March, 1983
175. Taber's Cyclopedic Medical Dictionary, 17th Ed., C.L.Thomas M.D., M.P.H., Ed., F.A. Davis Co., Philadelphia, 1993 p 1248
176. Palkiewicz, Pawel, et al."ADP-Ribosylation of Brain Neuronal Protiens Is Altered by In Vitro and In Vivo Exposure to Inorganic Mercury", *J Neurochemistry* 62: (5) pp2049-2052, 1994

177. Hunter,D., et al. "Poisoning by methyl-mercury compounds" *Quart J Med* 9:193-213, 1940
178. Hook, O., et al. "On alkyl mercury poisoning" *Acta Med Scand,* 150: 131-137, 1954
179. Lundgren, K.D. and Swensson, A., "Occupational poisoning by alkyl mercury compounds", *J Ind Hyg and Toxicol* 31:190-200, 1949
180. Siblerud, R.L., "A Comparison of mental health of multiple sclerosis patients with silver/mercury dental fillings and those with fillings removed", *Psychological Reports,* 70:1139-1151, 1992
181. Siblerud, R.L. and Keinholz, "Evidence that mercury from silver dental fillings may be an etiologic factor in multiple sclerosis", *The Science of the Total Environment,* 142:191-205, 1994
182. Ibid.
183. Ferris, E.B. and Fong, E., 2nd ed., Microbiology for health careers, Delmar Publishers, Inc., p 2, 1982
184. Janiki, K., et al. Correlation between contamination of the rural environment with mercury and occurrence of leukemia in men and cattle", *Chemosphere* 16:253-257, 1987
185. Duesburg, peter H. "AIDS epidemiology: Inconsistencies with human immunodeficiency virus and with ingectious disease," *Proc. Natl. Acad. Sci. USA* 88:1575-1579, Feb. 1991
186. Duesberg, Peter H. "AIDS acquired by drug consumption and other noncontagious risk factors," *Pharmac. Ther.* 55:201-277 1992
187. Taber's Cyclopedic Medical Dictionary, 17th Ed., C.L.Thomas M.D., M.P.H., Ed., F.A. Davis Co., Philadelphia, 1993 p 179

188. The Merck Manual of Diagnosis and Therapy, 16th Ed. R. Berkow, M.D. Ed., Merck Research Labs., N.J. 1992, p 1512-1513

189. Barber, R.E.,"Inorganic mercury intoxication reminiscent of amyotrophic lateral sclerosis", *J Occup Med,* 20:667-669, 1978

190. Adams, C., Ziegler, D., and Lin, J., "Mercury intoxication simulating amyotrophic lateral sclerosis", *JAMA* 250:642-643

191. Taber's Cyclopedic Medical Dictionary, 17th Ed., C.L.Thomas M.D., M.P.H., Ed., F.A. Davis Co., Philadelphia, 1993, p 348

192. "Mercury, draft for public comment", United States Dept. of Health and Human Services, PHS Oct. 1992 p 21

193. Amin-Zaki, L. et al, "Methylmercury poisoning in the Iraqi suckling infant: A longitudinal study over five years", *J App Toxicol,* 1(4): 210-214, 1981

194. Elhassani, S.B., "The many faces of methylmercury poisoning", *J Toxicol Clin Toxicol,* 19(8): 875-906, 1983

195. Trakhtenberg, I.M., Chronic effects of mercury on organisms, US dept. of Health Education and Welfare, Public Health Service, National Institutes of Health. DHEW Pub. No. (NIH) 74-473, USGPO, Wash D.C., 1974

196. Mercury, draft for public comment, United States Dept. of Health and Human Services, PHS Oct. 1992, p 21-23

197. Hanninen, H., "Behavior effects of occupational exposure to mercury and lead", *Acta Neurol Scand* 66:167-175, 1982

198. Miller,J., et al, "Subclinical psychomotor and neuromuscular changes in workers exposed to inorganic mercury", *Am Ind Hyg Assoc J* :724-733 1975

199. Goldstein, N., et al. "Metal neuropathy" in: Dyck, P., Thomas, P., Lambert, E., eds. Peripheral Neuropathy, Philadelphia, PA: W.B. Saunders, 1249-1251, 1975

200. Iyer, K., et al. "Mercury poisoning in a dentist", *Arch Neurol* 33:788-790, 1976

201. Shapiro, I.M., et al. "Neurophysiological and neuropsychological function in mercury exposed dentists" *Lancet* i:1147-1150, 1982

202. "Mercury toxicity in the dental office; a neglected problem" Mantyla, Donald G. and Wright, Orson D., *JADA* Vol.92 June 1976 p 1193

203. Taber's Cyclopedic Medical Dictionary, 17th Ed., C.L.Thomas M.D., M.P.H., Ed., F.A. Davis Co., Philadelphia, 1993, p76

204. Wenstrup, D., et al. "Trace element imbalances in isolated sub-cellular fractions of Alzheimer's disease brains", *Brain Research,* 553:125-131, 1990

205. Ehmann, W.E., et al. *Biol Trace Elem Res* 13:19-33, 1987

206. Ehmann, W.D., et al. "Brain trace element analysis instrumental NNA", *Neurotoxicology,* 7:197-206, 1976

207. Duhr, E., et al. FASEB 75th Annual Meeting, Atlanta, GA, April 21-25, 1991, Abstract # 493

208. Challem, J.J., and Lewin, R., "Beating Alzheimer's Disease: How Tom Warren Cured Himself", *Let's Live,* pp 56-59, June 1990

209. Ross, W.D. and Sholiton, M.C., "Specificity of psychiatric manifestations in relation to neurotoxic chemicals", *Acta Phychiat Scand,* 67 suppl 303:100-104, 1983

210. Gowdy, J.M. and Demers, F.X., "Whole blood mercury levels in mental hospital patients", *Am J Psychiatry,* 135(1):115-117, 1978

211. Piikivi, L. and Hanninen, H. "Subjective symptoms and psychological per-

formance of chlorine-alkalai workers", *Scand J Work Environ Health* 15(1):69-74, 1989

212. Maurissen, J.P.J., "History of mercury and mercurialism", *NY State J Med,* 81:1905, 1981

213. U.S. Dept. of Labor, Occupational Safety and Health Administration, August 1975, Job Health Hazards Series, "Mercury" OSHA 2234

214. Weiss, B., "Behavioral toxicology and environmental health science. Opportunity and challenge for psychology", *Am Psychologist,* Nov. 1983 pp 1174-1187

215. Blachly, P.H., Osterud, H.T., and Josslin, R., "Suicide in professional groups", *New Eng J Med,* 268:1278-1282, 1963

216. Foulds, D., et al. "Mercury poisoning and acrodynia", *Am J Dis Children* 141: 124-125, 1987

217. Sexton, D., et al. "A nonoccupational outbreak of inorganic mercury vapor poisoning" *Arch Environ Health* 33:186-191, 1976

218. Bourgeois, M., et al. "Mercury intoxication after topical application of a metallic mercury ointment", *Dermatologica* 172:48-51, 1986

219. Atkinson, W.S. "A colored reflex from the anterior capsule of the lens which occurs in mercurialism", *Am J Ophthal* 26:685-688, 1943

220. Bidstrup, P. et al. "Chronic mercury poisoning in men repairing direct current meters", *Lancet :* 856-861, 1951

221. Locket, S. and Nazaroo, I. "Eye changes following exposure to metallic mercury", *Lancet :* 528-530, 1952

222. Arons, I.J., "Care Products (contact lens)", *Optom. Management,* 15:45-53, 1979

223. Wilson L.A., Mcnatt J., Reitshell, R. , "Delayed Hypersensitivity to thimerosal in soft contact lens wearers", *Ophthalmology* (Rochester), 88:804-809, 1981

224. Mercury, draft for public comment, United States Dept. of Health and Human Services, PHS p. 18, Oct. 1992

225. *Weekly World News,* November 23, 1993

226. Queen, H.L., Chronic Mercury Toxicity. New hope against an Endemic Disease, Queen and Co. Health Communications, inc. , Colorado Springs, CO p 2, 1988

227. Veien, N.K., "Stomatitis and systemic dermatitis from mercury in amalgam dental restorations", *Dermatol Clin* 8(1):157-160, 1990

228. Brown, I.A., "Chronic mercurialism: A cause of the clinical syndrome of amyotrophic lateral sclerosis", *Arch Neurol Psychiatry* 72:674-681, 1954

229. Hallee, T.J.,"Diffuse lung disease caused by inhalation of mercury vapor", *Am Rev Respir Dis,* 99:430-436, 1969

230. Lilis, R. et al. "Acute mercury poisoning with severe chronic pulmonary manifestations", *Chest* 88:306-309, 1985

231. McFarland, R. and Reigel, H., "Chronic mercury poisoning from a single brief exposure", *J Occup Med* 20: 534, 1978

232. Sexton, D., et al. "A nonoccupational outbreak of inorganic mercury vapor poisoning" *Arch Environ Health* 33: 186-191, 1976

233. Snodgrass, W. et al. "Mercury poisoning from home gold ore processing: Use of penicillamine and dimercaprol", *JAMA* 246:1929-1931, 1981

234. Cook and Yates, "Fatal mercury intoxication of a dental surgery assistant", *Brit Dent J* 127(12):553-555, 1969

235. Boyd, N.D. et al. "Mercury from dental 'silver' tooth fillings impairs sheep kidney function", *The American Physiological Society* R1010-R1014, 1991

236. Hahn, L.J., et al. "Whole body imaging of the distribution of mercury released from dental fillings into monkey tissues", *The FASEB Journal* Vol. 4:3256-3260 Nov. 1990

237. Goodman and Gilman, The Pharmacological Basis of Therapeutics, 6th ed. Macmillan Pub. Co. Inc., N.Y. 1980

238. Occupational Exposure to Inorganic Mercury, OSHA, 1973

239. Buchet, J., et al., "Assessment of renal function of workers exposed to inorganic lead, cadmium, or mercury vapor", *J Occup Med*, 22:741-750, 1980

240. The Merck Manual of Diagnosis and Therapy, 16th Ed. R. Berkow, M.D. Ed., Merck Research Labs., N.J. 1992

241. Ibid

242. Lee, Min-Wei, "Two studies suggest risk from silver fillings", *Chicago Tribune*, Wed. August 15,1990

243. Campbell, J., "Acute mercurial poisoning by inhalation of mercury vapor in an infant", *Can Med Assoc J* 58:72-75, 1948

244. Kanluen, S. and Gottlieb, C.A., "A clinical pathologic study of four adult cases of acute mercury inhalation toxicity", *Arch Pathol Lab Med*, 115(1):56-60, 1991

245. Matthes, F., et al. "Acute poisoning associated with inhalation of mercury vapor: Report of four cases", *Pediatrics*, 22: 675-688, 1958

246. McFarland, R. and Reigel, H., "Chronic mercury poisoning from a single brief exposure", *J Occup Med* 20:534, 1978

247. Milne, J., et al. "Acute mercurial pneumonitis" *Br J Ind Med*, 27:334-338, 1970

248. Teng, C. and Brennan, J., "Acute mercury vapor poisoning: A report of four cases with radiographic and pathologic correlation", *Radiology*, 73:354-361, 1959

249. Goodman and Gilman, The Pharmacological Basis of Therapeutics, 6th ed. Macmillan Pub. Co. Inc., N.Y. 1980

250. Campbell, J., "Acute mercurial poisoning by inhalation of mercury vapor in an infant", *Can Med Assoc J* 58:72-75, 1948

251. Kanluen, S. and Gottlieb, C.A., "A clinical pathologic study of four adult cases of acute mercury inhalation toxicity", *Arch Pathol Lab Med*, 115(1):56-60, 1991

252. Teng, C. and Brennan, J., "Acute mercury vapor poisoning: A report of four cases with radiographic and pathologic correlation", *Radiology*, 73:354-361, 1959

253. Walleczek, Jan, "Bioelectromagnetics and the Question of 'Subtle Energies'", *Noetic Sciences Review*, 28:33-36, Winter 1993

254. Ibid

255. Engley, F.B., Jr., "Evaluation of Mercury Compounds as Antiseptics," *Annals of the New York Academy of Sciences*, 53:197-206, 1950

256. Federal Register, Vol. 47, No. 2 Tuesday, January 5, 1982, p 441

257. Miller, N.Z., "Vaccines and Natural Health", *Mothering*, 70:44-53, Spring 1994

258. Ibid

259. Ibid

260. Ibid

261. Miller, N.Z., "Vaccines and Natural Health", *Mothering*, 70:44-53, Spring 1994

262. Physician's Desk Reference, 47th Ed., Medical Economics Data, Oradell, N.J., 1993

263. Taber's Cyclopedic Medical Dictionary, 17th Ed., C.L.Thomas M.D., M.P.H., Ed., F.A. Davis Co., Philadelphia, 1993, p 1283

264. Physician's Desk Reference, 47th Ed., Medical Economics Data, Oradell, N.J., 1993

265. Miller, N.Z., "Vaccines and Natural

Health", *Mothering*, 70:44-53, Spring 1994
266. Ibid
267. Physician's Desk Reference, 47th Ed., Medical Economics Data, Oradell, N.J., 1993
268. Miller, N.Z., "Vaccines and Natural Health", *Mothering*, 70:44-53, Spring 1994
269. Physician's Desk Reference, 47th Ed., Medical Economics Data, Oradell, N.J., 1993
270. Chopra, M.D., Deepak, Ageless Body, Timeless Mind, Harmony Books, N.Y. 1993 p 9
271. Monte, Tom "Fear and Loathing in the Dentist's Chair" *Natural Health Magazine*, July/August 1992 p 68 Reprinted with permission from *Natural Health Magazine* For a free trial issue call 1-800-925-3330
272. Denton, M.D., Sandra "The Mercury Cover-Up" *Sarasota ECO Report* Vol. 3 No. 5 May, 1993 p 1
273. Knight, A.L.: "Mercury and its compounds", Occupational Medicine: Principles and Practical Applications, Zenz, C., Ed., Chicago, Illinois, Year Book Medical Publishers, 1975, p 668
274. Ramazzini, B.: De Morbis Artificum Bernardini Ramazzini Diatriba, 1713, translated by W.C Wright, Chicago, Illinois, The University of Chicago Press, 1940, p50
274a. Fax transmittal from D. Carrington of the Environmental Protection Department of Orange County, Florida on 6/6/95 *"Drinking water standard, monitoring and reporting"* DEP 62-550 [Reference: 62-550.310(1)(a)] from the REGfiles, inc., Tallahassee, Florida 1995.
275. Nebergall, Schmidt and Holtzclaw, General Chemistry, fourth ed., D.C. Heath and Co., 1972
276. *Morbidity and Mortality Weekly Reports;* NE J Med, Publishers, Vol. 40 No. 23 June

14, 1991
277. Nash, Kent D. and Bentley, John E. "Is Restorative Dentistry on its way Out?", *JADA* Vol. 122 No.9 August 1991 p 79
278. Svare, C.W., et al, "Dental amalgam : a potential source of mercury vapor exposure", *J Dent Res,* 59 Special issue A: p341, abstract 293, 1980
279. Hirshfeld, Neal "The Poison Plant, Mercury and Madness at Brooklyn's Pymm Thermometer factory", *New York Daily News Magazine* March 15, 1987 pp 22-25
280. Hemenway, Caroline G. "Amalgam Declared Hazardous", *Dentistry Today,* Feb. 1989. p 10 Reprinted by permission of *Dentistry Today*
281. Ibid
282. Hemenway, Caroline G. "Dentists to Pay for Mercury Cleanup", *Dentistry Today,* Oct. 1988 p12 Reprinted by permission of *Dentistry Today*
283. Hemenway, Caroline G. "Dentists to Pay for Mercury Cleanup", *Dentistry Today,* Oct. 1988 p 55 Reprinted by permission of *Dentistry Today*
284. Ibid
285. Federal Register, Vol. 47, No. 2 Tuesday, January 5, 1982 p 440-441
286. Arons, I.J. "Care Products (contact lens)" *Optom. Management* 1979;15:45-53
287. Wilson L.A., Mcnatt J., Reitshell, R.; Delayed "Hypersensitivity to thimerosal in soft contact lens wearers" *Ophthalmology* (Rochester) 1981; 88:804-809
288. *Mercury-free News,* May, 1992 p 6
289. *International DAMS Newsletter* Vol. IV, Issue 2, Spring, 1994 p 2
290. Taber's Cyclopedic Medical Dictionary, 17th Ed., C.L.Thomas M.D., M.P.H., Ed., F.A. Davis Co., Philadelphia, 1993 pp939-940, 1786
291.White, R.R. and Brandt, R.L. "Develop-

ment of mercury hypersensitivity among dental students", *JADA* Vol. 92 June 1976. p. 1206 Reprinted by permission of the ADA Publishing Co., Inc.

292. Vandengerge, J., Moodie, A.S. and Keller, Jr., R.E. "Blood serum mercury test report", *JADA* Vol. 94, June 1977 pp 1156 Reprinted by permission of the ADA Publishing Co., Inc.

293. U.S. Dept. of Labor, Occupational Safety and Health Administration, August 1975, Job Health Hazards Series, "Mercury" OSHA 2234

294. Ibid

294a. Metlen, Richard, D.D.S., "Mercury spills and spills and their subsequent sequelae," *CDA Journal,* February 1984 pp 33-35.

295. Miller, S.L.et al."Mercury vapor levels in the dental office: a survey" *JADA* Vol.89, No.5, Nov.1974 pp1084-1091 Reprinted by Permission of the ADA Publishing Co., Inc.

296. Ibid

297. "Metal, Chemical Hazards rampant in dental offices." *Florida Environments,* July 1993, p 19 Reprinted by permission of *Florida Environments*

298. U.S. Government Printing office Document entitled "Mercury" Occupational Safety and Health Administration, August 1975 OSHA 2234

299. Trakhtenberg, I.M., <u>Chronic effects of mercury on organisms,</u> US dept. of Health Education and Welfare, Public Health Service, National Institutes of Health. DHEW Pub. No. (NIH) 74-473, USGPO, Wash D.C., 1974

300. "Metal, Chemical Hazards rampant in dental offices." *Florida Environments,* July 1993, p 19 Reprinted by permission of *Florida Environments*

301. McNerney, Richard T and McNerney, John J. "A Review. Mercury Contamination In the Dental Office" , *NYS Dental Journal,* Nov. 1979, p 457

302. Council on Dental Materials, Instruments and Equipment "Recommendations in mercury hygiene, 1984", *JADA* Vol. 109 Oct. 1984 p 617 Reprinted by permission of ADA Publishing Co., Inc.

303. Ross,W.D. and Sholiton, M.C., "Specificity of psychiatric manifestations in relation to neurotoxic chemicals", *Acta Phychiat Scand,* 67, Suppl. 303:100-104, 1983

304. Stock, A. and Jaensch, E., Translation by Mats Hanson, "Nothing new under the sun: Experiences with mercury poisoning related by Dr. Alfred Stock and Dr. E. Jaensch in 1926" *J Orthomol Psych,* Vol. 12 No. 3:202-207, 1983

305. Triebig, G. and Schaller, K. H. "Neurotoxic effects in mercury-exposed workers", *Neurobehav Toxicol Teratol,* Vol. 4 No. 6:717-720, 1982

306. Gowdy, J. M. and Demers, F.X., "Whole blood mercury levels in mental hospital patients", *AM J Psychiatry,* 135 (1):115-117, 1978

307. "Metal, Chemical Hazards rampant in dental offices." *Florida Environments,* July 1993, p 19 Reprinted by permission of *Florida Environments*

308. McCann, Daniel, "Another Regulation? State and local Officials scrutinizing amalgam waste in water supplies" *ADA News,* Vol. 25 No. 4 February 21, 1994, p 1-13 Reprinted by permission of ADA Publishing Co., Inc.

309. Ibid

310. Ibid

311. Ibid

312. Environmental Dental Association, letter of 7/27/92 titled "Environmental Experts Issue Warning on Mercury Poisoning 'Only A Matter of Time Before It Reaches Top of Food

Chain'" p 2
313. Ibid
314. World Health Organization, 1991; *Environmental Health Criteria 118, Organic Mercury.* WHO, Geneva
315. *Mercury-Free News* May 1992, p 14
316. Shanklin, Mary "What we flush may come back to haunt us" *The Orlando Sentinel,* Monday, Dec. 7,1992, pp A-1 to A-10
317. "Metal, chemical hazards rampant in dental offices" *Florida Environments* July, 1993. p 19
318. Clarke, David "Let Them Drink Wastewater" *Garbage,* Summer 1994 " pp 10-12
318a. Fax transmittal from D. Carrington of the Environmental Protection Department of Orange County, Florida 6/6/95 "Drinking water standard, monitoring and reporting" DEP 62-550 [Reference: 62-550.310(1)(a)] from the REGfiles, inc., Tallahassee, Florida 1995.
319. Clarke, David *"Let Them Drink Wastewater" Garbage,* Summer 1994 " pp 10-12
319a. Deneen, Sally "Our Endangered Everglades" *E Magazine,* Vol. III No. 6 Nov./Dec. 1992 pp 20-22 Reprinted with permission from *E Magazine*
319aa. Skare, I and Engqvist, A. , "Human Exposure to mercury and silver released from dental amalgam restorations" *Arch of Envir Health* Vol. pp 384-394 1994
320. Ibid
321. Ibid
322. Royals, Homer and Lange, Ted "Mercury in Florida Fish and Wildlife" *Florida Wildlife,* March-April 1990, pp 3-6
323. Deneen, Sally "Our Endangered Everglades" *E Magazine,* Vol. III No. 6 Nov./Dec. 1992 pp 20-22 Reprinted with permission from *E Magazine*

324. Assoc. Press "Mercury levels continue to go up in Everglades" *The Orlando Sentinel,* Tues. July 21 ,1992 p B-5
325. Ibid
326. Ibid
327. Assoc. Press "Study: Mercury-tainted fish is a widespread problem" *The Orlando Sentinel,* Thurs. Sept. 3, 1992 p A-16
328. Ibid
329. Beasley, Alex and Glisch, John "How much more poison has yet to surface?" *The Orlando Sentinel* Sunday, Dec. 13, 1992
330. "Does Your Patient Have a Mercury Problem?" *Mercury - Free News,* Vol. 5 No. 1 Jan. 1992 p 1
330a. Harada, Masazumi, M.D. with Aileen Smith, *Minamata Disease: A Medical Report* in the book Minamata, words and photographs by Eugene Smith and Aileen Smith p 180
331. "Florida Health Advisory - Mercury in Florida Freshwater Fish" Produced by the Florida Dept. of HRS 6/93
332. "Does Your Patient Have a Mercury Problem?" *Mercury - Free News,* Vol. 5 No. 1 Jan. 1992 p 2
333. Ibid
334. *Mercury-Free News,* May 1992, p 14
335. Ibid
336. Ibid
337. "Does Your Patient Have a Mercury Problem?" *Mercury-Free News* Vol. 5 No.1 January 1992 p 2
338. Harada, Masazumi, M.D. with Aileen Smith, *Minamata Disease: A Medical Report* in the book Minamata, words and photographs by Eugene Smith and Aileen Smith p 183
339. Tedeschi, L.G., "The Minamata disease", *Am J Forensic Med Pathol,* 3(4): 335-338, 1982
340. Harada, M., "Congenital Minamata disease: Intrauterine methylmercury poisoning." *Teratology,* 18 (2):285-288, 1978
341. Queen, H.L., Chronic Mercury Toxicity,

New Hope Against an Endemic Disease, Queen and Co. Health Communications, inc. Colorado Sprgs, CO, 1988 p 17-18

342. Eyl,Thomas B. "Organic-Mercury Food Poisoning", *NE J Med* April 1, 1971, pp 706-709

343. Ibid

344. Royals, Homer and Lange, Ted "Mercury in Florida Fish and Wildlife", *Florida Wildlife* March-April 1990 p 4

345. Eyl,Thomas B. "Organic-Mercury Food Poisoning", *NE J Med* April 1, 1971, p. 706-709

346. Ibid

347. Ibid

348. *CRA Newsletter* Vol. 18, Issue 5, May 1994

349. Nash, Kent D. and Bentley, John E. "Is Restorative Dentistry on its way Out?", *JADA* Vol. 122 No.9 August 1991 p 79

350. Regan, Mary Beth "Don't gloss over mercury paint labels" *The Orlando Sentinel,* Friday, October 19,1990 , p D-5

350a. Anderson, Penny Elliot, Senior Ed. "Dental fees keep pace with low inflation rate" *Dental Economics* p 37 May 1995

351. Meier, Barry "Government Bans Mercury in Interior Latex Paints" *The New York Times,* Saturday, June 30, 1990

352. Chen, Edwin "Mercury Use in Paints to be Curbed" *The Orlando Sentinel,* Thursday, October 18, 1990

353. "Latex Paint may be peril to Children" compiled from wire reports *The Orlando Sentinel,* Thursday, October 18, 1990

354. Environmental Dental Association, letter of 7/27/92 titled "Environmental Experts Issue Warning on Mercury Poisoning 'Only A Matter of Time Before It Reaches Top of Food Chain" p 2

354a. Confirmed on phone by Dennis Nester with the Orange County Environment Protection department (407) 836-7400 on 7/5/95

355. "Dangerous when dead-Bad news from teeth" *Newsweek,* August 27,1990 p 55

355a. Anderson, Penny Elliot, Senior Ed. "Dental fees keep pace with low inflation rate" *Dental Economics* p 37 May 1995

356. *International DAMS Newsletter,* Spring 1994 p 2

357. *International DAMS Newsletter,* Spring 1994 p 2,8

358. IAOMT President's Message ; letter sent out with the *In-Vivo* IAOMT Newsletter of June 1994 written by Dr. David C. Kennedy, President, IAOMT

359. "Warning labels placed on dental filling packaging" *Health Advocate,* Houston Enterprises, Inc. Phoenix AZ. Feb. 1994 p 4

360. "Consumer Warnings Overruled" *International DAMS Newsletter,* Vol. IV:4 p11 Fall, 1994

361. *Mercury-Free News,* May, 1992 p 6

362. Aposhian, H.V., et al. "Urinary mercury after administration of DMPS: correlation with dental amalgam score", *FASEB J.* 6:2472-2476, 1992

363. Friberg, L., ed. *Environmental Health Criteria, Vol. 118:* Inorganic Mercury, p 36 World Health Organization, Geneva 1991

364. Inasmasu, T. et al. "Mercury concentration change in human hair after the ingestion of canned tuna fish", *Bull Environ Contam Toxicol* 41(4): 508-514, 1986

365. Vimy, M.J. and Lorschieder, F.L. "Dental amalgam mercury daily dose estimated from intra-oral vapor measurements: A predictor of mercury accumulation in human tissues" *J Trace Elem Exper Med* 3:111-113, 1990

366. *Clinical Research Associates Newsletter,* Vol. 18, issue 5, May, 1994 p 1

INDEX

251

255

paint, mercury in, 197
Pakistan, 194
panic attacks, 24
parasites, 106
paste, silver, 46
patch testing, 226
patient drape, 227
penicillamine, 112, 139
penicillin, 119
periodontics, 136
periodontitis, 136-138
peripheral nervous system, 125
personality changes, 80, 132
pertussis, 146-147
phenylmercuric nitrate, 163
physician-dentists, 56
pituitary gland, 98, 99
plasma, 105
platelets, 105, 106
Pliny the Elder, 44
pneumonitis, 64
Podgor, Joe, 185
Poison Control Center, 172
poisoning, mercury, ii, 6, 63
polio vaccine, 148
    inactivated, 149
    live oral, 149
Popular Science, 166
potable reuse, 184
pregnancy, 17, 101
preservatives, 146
    mercury-based, 21, 146
proteins, 105
psychologic, 123
psychological
    problems, 24
    symptoms, 32, 228

Q
Question Authority, 223
quicksilver, 86

R
radioactive isotopes, 202
radio stations, picking up, 144
rashes, 24
rectal bleeding, 103
recurrent decay, 79
red mercuric sulfide, 189
refined sugar intake, 12
reflexes, slow, 95
Regnart, Louis, 45
renal, 138-140
reproductive disorders, 93-94
respiratory, 140
    complications, 78
Reye's Syndrome, 149
rheumatoid arthritis, 28, 104, 106, 110-
    114, 121
ringing in the ears, 144, 228
Rocky Mountain Research Institute, 116
root canal therapy, 79
Royal Mineral Succedaneum, 49
rubber dam, 227
rubella vaccine, 148, 149

S
salivation, excessive, 136
scrap amalgam, 201
sectioning the fillings, 227
Segel, Dr. Bernie, 219
selenium blocks, 208
self control, loss of, 124
self-confidence, 124
self-image, 14
sensitive eyes, 135
sensory disturbances, 18
sequential removal, 227-229
short term memory loss, 6, 27, 28
shyness, 6, 124
sick teeth, 13
Silent Spring, 217
silver fillings, i, ii, 3, 52, 56, 89, 92, ...
silver paste, 46

Order Form

Please send ____ copies of <u>MERCURY FREE...the</u>

<u>wisdom behind the global consumer movement to</u>

<u>ban "silver" dental fillings</u> to:

Name: _____
(Please print)

Address: _____
(Street & Number)

_____
(City, State, Zip or Province & Mail Code)

Phone: (_____)_____

Signature _____ Date:_____

Cost is $16.95 plus $3.95 shipping and handling each.
In CANADA, cost is $18.95 plus $4.95 shipping and
handling. In U.S. or Canada call 800/266-5564 (24 hrs)
for up to 40% discount on multiple orders.
FL residents add 6% sales tax.

☐ Enclosed is a check payable to STCS Distributors,
Box 246, Dept. BK, Glassboro, NJ 08028-0246.
(Expect delivery in seven working days.)

☐ I am faxing my order to 609/881-8042,(24hrs) or will
phone toll-free to 800/266-5564 (24hrs). My_____
Credit Card # _____ expires __/__/__
(Expect delivery in five to seven working days.)

International orders (outside U.S. or Canada),
call 609/863-1014 (24-hrs); or FAX your order
609/881-8042 (24 hrs).
E-MAIL: stcsbook@aol.com